28-Day Mediterranean Diet
Heart-Healthy Solution

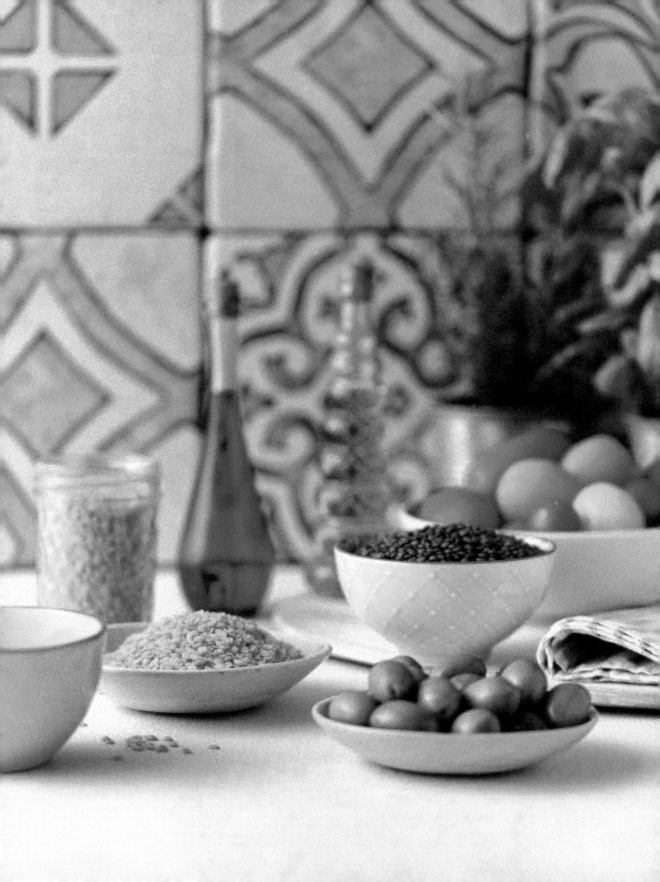

28-Day
Mediterranean Diet
Heart-Healthy Solution

The Pesco-Mediterranean Plan
for Optimal Heart Health

Lauren O'Connor, MS, RDN

ROCKRIDGE
PRESS

As of press time, the URLs in this book link or refer to existing websites on the internet. Rockridge Press is not responsible for the outdated, inaccurate, or incomplete content available on these sites.

Copyright © 2022 by Rockridge Press

All rights reserved. No part of this publication may be reproduced, stored in a retrieval system, or transmitted in any form or by any means, electronic, mechanical, photocopying, recording, scanning, or otherwise without the prior written permission of the Publisher. Requests to the Publisher for permission should be addressed to the Permissions Department, Rockridge Press, 1955 Broadway, Suite 400, Oakland, CA 94612.

First Rockridge Press trade paperback edition June 2022

Rockridge Press and the Rockridge Press logo are trademarks or registered trademarks of Callisto Media Inc. and/or its affiliates in the United States and other countries and may not be used without written permission.

For general information on our other products and services, please contact our Customer Care Department within the United States at (866) 744-2665, or outside the United States at (510) 253-0500.

Some of the recipes originally appeared, in different form, in *Essential Ketogenic Mediterranean Diet Cookbook, The Big Book of Mediterranean Diet Cooking, The Easy 5-Ingredient Pescatarian Cookbook, The Easy Mediterranean Diet Meal Plan, The 5-Ingredient Mediterranean Cookbook, One-Pot Mediterranean Diet, 14-Day Mediterranean Diet Plan for Beginners, The 28-Day DASH Diet Weight Loss Plan, The Pescatarian Cookbook,* and *The Truly Healthy Pescatarian Cookbook.*

Paperback ISBN: 978-1-63878-868-3 | eBook ISBN: 979-8-88608-114-5

Manufactured in the United States of America

Interior and Cover Designer: Linda Kocur
Art Producer: Samantha Ulban
Editor: Marjorie DeWitt
Production Editor: Emily Sheehan
Production Manager: David Zapanta

Photography © Nadine Greeff, Cover and pp. vi, 142; Darren Muir, pp. ii, x, 16, 52, 77, 84, 101, 118; Thomas J. Story, pp. 35, 49, 56, 63, 66, 130, 136; Evi Abeler, p. 36; Marija Vidal, p. 43, 96; Annie Martin, p. 80; All other images used under license Shutterstock.

Author photo courtesy of Bridie Macdonald

10 9 8 7 6 5 4 3 2 1

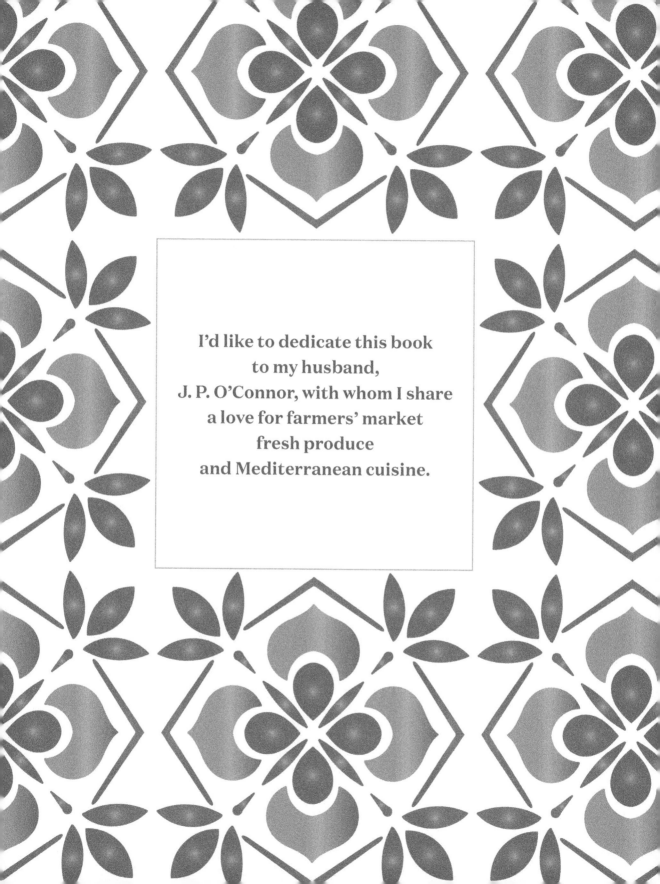

I'd like to dedicate this book
to my husband,
J. P. O'Connor, with whom I share
a love for farmers' market
fresh produce
and Mediterranean cuisine.

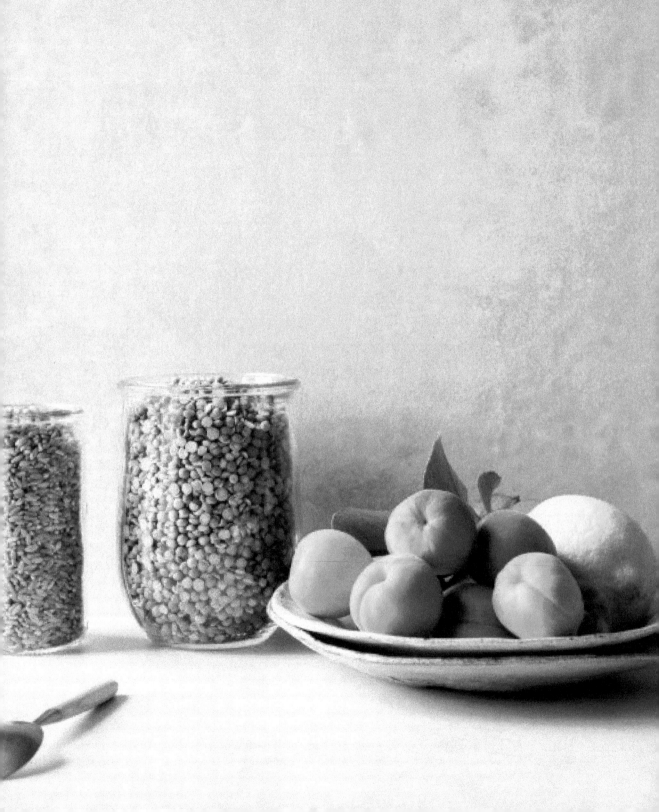

Contents

Introduction

Congratulations on choosing to follow the Mediterranean diet on your journey to heart health. Having guidance to seek out healthy foods and prepare delicious, nutritious meals can make this shift both attainable and sustainable. In this cookbook, you can expect to see a variety of recipes with common, easy-to-find ingredients and a 28-day meal plan to kick-start and simplify your new, heart-healthy way of eating.

The Mediterranean diet is an all-around healthy diet that has been recommended for years by doctors and dietitians alike. As you'll read more about in the next chapter, research indicates that the optimal diet for heart health is a pescatarian version of the Mediterranean diet, rich in vegetables, fruits, healthy fats, and seafood-based proteins. This cookbook adopts that approach, and its goal is to help you implement it in your life. While it is important to find the right balance of foods that work for you, in these pages you won't find any recipes that call for poultry or meat.

To be honest, I can devour a vibrant bowl of veggies, and I prefer fish over poultry or beef. But I didn't always love seafood. The mere exceptions were smoked salmon (lox and bagels) and tuna fish. A 1970s child (to non-hippie parents), I was accustomed to TV dinners, SPAM, and Tang. And veggies were few and far between, if you don't count peas and potatoes.

Leaving the nest in my college years, I explored healthier options because I wanted to become more fit. But the greatest contribution to my heart-healthy lifestyle is my husband. He was a huge influence on my tastes and culinary adventures when we were dating in my mid-twenties.

My husband (then boyfriend) would regularly shop the local farmers' market to buy a fresh catch from the fishmonger and an array of in-season veggies—colorful plant foods that kept our dinners healthy, vibrant, and tasty. The result was always divine. Cooking alongside him was my true introduction to healthy living and a precursor to my occupation as a culinary dietitian.

Like me, people come to healthy diets for several reasons, and it may happen at various times in their lives. Whether you are cooking for a loved one with a heart condition or are proactively seeking to adopt a heart-healthy diet for yourself, pursuing a wholesome, nutritionally sound lifestyle is within your reach. I hope this book helps you not only embrace a heart-healthy way of eating but also enjoy many delicious meals to come.

Chapter 1

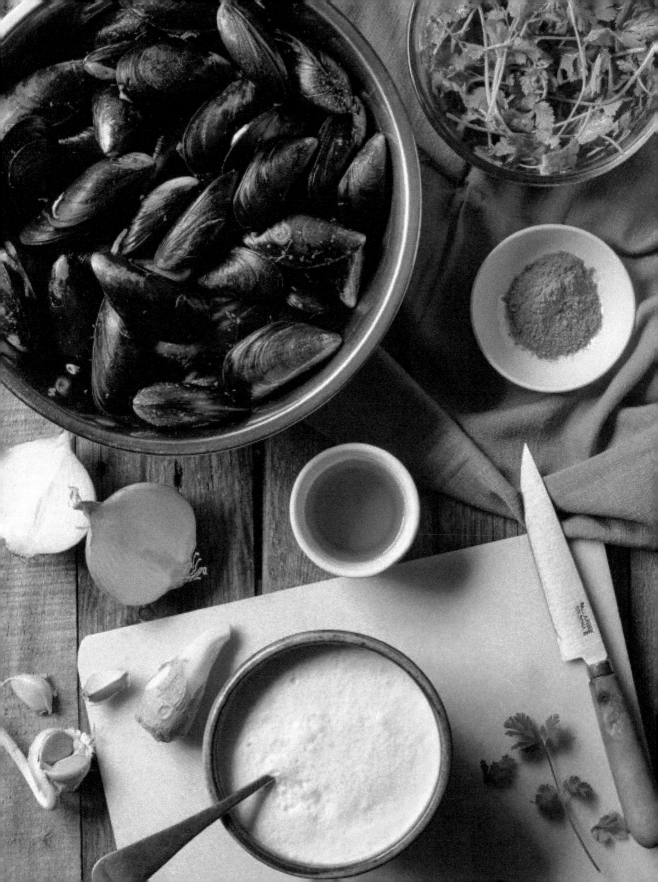

The Mediterranean Diet for Heart Health

If you are looking for ways to manage your cholesterol, lower your sodium intake, and still enjoy flavorful meals, you've come to the right place. This chapter explains the why and how of following a pescatarian version of the Mediterranean diet to develop a heart-healthy lifestyle you can maintain.

Making Fresh Choices for Your Health

The Mediterranean diet has long been considered the gold standard for heart health. With its roots in Spain, France, Italy, Greece, Turkey, Israel, Morocco, Libya, Lebanon, Algeria, Tunisia, and Egypt, it highlights colorful, flavorful, plant-rich cuisine. Though food staples and dishes vary from one Mediterranean region to another, the style of diet emphasizes the intake of fruits, vegetables, whole grains, and lean proteins.

The Mediterranean diet, which has existed for centuries, has gained popularity over the past few decades for its health benefits, emphasis on bold flavors, and simplicity of preparation. Focusing on freshly sourced foods, the Mediterranean diet supports the ideals of a booming farm-to-table movement to promote more food security, food sustainability, and self-reliant communities. We've heard terms like "plant-centric" and "plant-forward" become more mainstream over the past several years.

The Pesco-Mediterranean Approach

Current research, including the findings of a much-cited study published in the *Journal of the American College of Cardiology*, suggests that a pescatarian version of the Mediterranean diet (pesco-Mediterranean) is optimal for lowering the risk of heart disease and promoting general good health. A pesco-Mediterranean diet emphasizes seafood as its primary source of animal protein along with some dairy and eggs.

While there's plenty of research supporting the benefits of the plant-rich vegan diet, nutrient deficiencies may be of concern. Without animal protein, it can be challenging to get enough vitamins B_{12} and D, calcium, iron, zinc, iodine, omega-3 fatty acids, and protein. On the other hand, science has repeatedly shown that diets heavy in animal proteins, particularly fatty red meats, can be detrimental to one's heart health.

The pesco-Mediterranean diet bridges the gap between vegan and non-vegan diets by including protein from seafood, dairy, and eggs. The recipes and meal plans in this book focus on this pesco-Mediterranean dietary plan to offer an effective and delicious approach to eating for optimal heart health.

Before diving into the recipes, let's learn how certain foods can benefit your heart and how other foods may harm it.

How Foods Help (and Hurt) Your Heart

If you think of your blood flow like a highway, you'll realize that it's important to keep it free from traffic jams so that it can deliver nutrients properly and when needed to the cells throughout your body. Your blood also transports oxygen, so good circulation is essential for ensuring that all your body's systems work in harmony for overall health.

Two key elements of a heart-healthy diet are eating foods that promote a smooth and steady blood flow through the cardiovascular pathway and minimizing those foods that impede that flow. The pesco-Mediterranean diet includes fruits, vegetables, whole grains, and fish—all of which help protect your arteries and promote healthy blood flow.

You may also visualize the circulatory system as a web of information where every entity in your body relies on proper signaling and response to send and receive messages needed to operate and function properly. An unhealthy diet can derail proper communications and affect metabolism (how the body converts food into energy) and heart health.

In a healthy individual, when blood sugars rise, the pancreas produces insulin—a hormone that signals cells to take in blood sugar. This enables the body to use or store those sugars for energy. However, when sugar intake is constantly high, the system can get out of whack. Over time, cells stop responding to the insulin, or become insulin resistant. The pancreas has to work harder to pump more insulin to trigger a cellular response. Eventually, the pancreas can't keep up with insulin production, and blood sugars continue to rise.

Hyperglycemia, or high blood sugar, weakens the elasticity of the blood vessels, causing them to narrow, which impedes the flow of blood. Not only does this affect the delivery of oxygen and nutrients to the body, but it can also lead to diabetes, high blood pressure, and, ultimately, cardiovascular complications.

The important thing to understand is that certain types of foods are more likely to have a negative impact on the body over time, increasing the risk for heart disease and stroke. Foods that are high in saturated fats can clog up the vessels and lead to a build-up of fatty deposits that affect the flow of blood. Sodium-rich foods may increase blood pressure, which makes the heart work harder. Sugar, refined carbohydrates, and alcohol increase triglycerides, high levels of which are linked to prediabetes and diabetes, which can increase the risk of heart disease and stroke.

By following the pesco-Mediterranean diet and using the recipes and meal plans in this book, you'll be consuming minimal and safe amounts of foods with those possibly harmful effects while predominantly eating foods that strengthen the arteries and promote healthy circulation by reducing fatty deposits and lowering blood pressure.

Five Dishes to Try First

I'm delighted to share that all the recipes in this cookbook deliver on the promise of healthy-meets-delicious. Here are some I think are particularly good as far as setting the stage for this diet.

Loaded Avocado Sweet Potato "Toast": A sweeter, lower-carb, and less processed version of traditional avocado toast, this breakfast offers plenty of dietary fiber. You'll get a healthy dose of heart-smart protein, too. While the protein comes mostly from egg whites, the egg yolks contain most of the nutrients found in eggs, including essential fatty acids (omega-3s), potassium, B-vitamins, iron, and vitamins A, D, and E. You can find this recipe in chapter 3 (page 42).

Shakshuka: A popular dish across the Mediterranean, shakshuka is a crowd-pleasing recipe with its zesty, hearty, tomato-rich blend. This dish includes a nice balance of herbs and spices as well as lycopene-rich tomatoes, onions, and bell peppers. You can find this veggie-packed egg recipe in chapter 3 (page 48).

Stuffed Cherry Tomatoes: These pop-in-your-mouth delights are simple to make, and they are a plant-centric appetizer with a combo of cucumber, red onion, and fresh basil in the mix. Protein-rich ricotta stuffed into cherry tomatoes makes this recipe fun and satisfying. You can find this appetizer in chapter 4 (page 62).

Fresh Gazpacho Soup: Cool and refreshing, this soup hails from Spanish cuisine. It's as tasty as it is simple with a blend of tomatoes, cucumbers, and garlic, and it is seasoned to perfection with vinegar, salt, and pepper. Simply blend the ingredients, and you've got yourself a tasty dish in practically no time at all. You can find this recipe in chapter 5 (page 81).

Mediterranean Snapper with Olives and Feta: This mild whitefish is complemented by the fragrant combo of traditional Greek staples—olives, tomatoes, feta, and garlic. From start to finish, this savory dish takes just thirty-five minutes to make. You can find this recipe in chapter 6 (page 113).

Heart Medications and Diet

There are certain dietary restrictions doctors recommend when a person is taking some of the most common heart medications. This is because certain foods can affect the impact of the drugs, which can lead to medical complications.

Statin Drugs: Common statins include Lipitor, Crestor, and Zocor. When you take these cholesterol-lowering statin drugs, it's important to avoid grapefruit because it can interfere with the liver's ability to process these medications, consequently causing a buildup of the drug in your system.

Blood Thinners: When taking Coumadin or Heparin, you'll want to watch your vitamin K intake. Vitamin K is a coagulant, which prevents you from bleeding, so it can reduce the effectiveness of blood thinners. Potassium may be contraindicated for Heparin because it may increase Heparin's side effects.

Blood Pressure Medications: These drugs include ACE Inhibitors, Arbs, Spironolactone, Labetalol, and Propranolol. Foods that contain furanocoumarins, such as citrus, block the enzyme that controls the length of time a medication is activated in your system. When a medication is active in the body longer than expected, it's possible for a person to overdose without knowing it. You may also have to watch your intake of potassium because ACE Inhibitors and Arbs may raise potassium levels. Too much potassium in the blood can lead to heart distress.

Check with your doctor or pharmacist if you are unclear about your medication and how it may react with the foods in your diet.

The Benefits of a Pesco-Mediterranean Diet

Scientists, doctors, and other health professionals value a pesco-Mediterranean diet as a sound solution to protecting heart health because as a plant-based whole foods diet with an emphasis on fish as its primary source of animal protein, it protects against cardiovascular disease (CVD) and the risk factors leading up to it.

Cardiovascular Disease

One of the key methods for promoting cardiovascular health is adhering to a whole foods diet rich in plants, nuts, seeds, whole grains, and legumes. These foods provide many of the essential nutrients we need without the excess saturated fats of highly processed foods, which are often full of sodium and added sugars. Including fish in the diet delivers high-quality protein as well as heart-protective vitamins B_{12} and D, two essential vitamins found more sparingly in vegan diets.

Diabetes

Studies have shown that a Mediterranean diet can reduce heightened HbA1C, a marker significant in the progression of diabetes and in cardiovascular risk. A 2015 systemic review published in *BMJ Open* covering eight meta-analyses and five randomized controlled trials concluded that adherence to the Mediterranean diet improved blood glucose levels and HbA1C values in people with type 2 diabetes. It also indicated lower risk for developing the disease. Additionally, the Mediterranean diet has been linked to lower incidence of central obesity (excess abdominal fat), a factor that contributes to insulin resistance and type 2 diabetes.

High Blood Pressure

The Dietary Approaches to Stop Hypertension (DASH) diet evolved from research and continues to be a safe and effective way to lower blood pressure. Like DASH, the pesco-Mediterranean diet emphasizes fruits and vegetables, whole grains, nuts, seeds, and the use of unsaturated oils. Potassium helps control high blood pressure. It also helps reduce tension within your blood vessel walls. The more potassium you eat, such as from fruits and vegetables, the more sodium you excrete via urine, according to a 2017 article in *Nutrients*. Lowering saturated fats through limited animal proteins is another commonality between DASH and the pesco-Mediterranean diet. While the Mediterranean diet doesn't specifically limit sodium, a plant-based whole foods diet helps reduce excess sodium consumption as sodium is "hidden" in many highly processed foods.

High Cholesterol

According to a 2019 article in *Molecular Nutrition & Food Research*, increasing the consumption of nuts, legumes, whole grains, extra-virgin olive oil, and fish promotes HDL (good cholesterol) function for improved cardiovascular health. The pesco-Mediterranean diet, with its whole foods plant-based approach, includes such foods. Furthermore, it emphasizes the use of extra-virgin olive oil (over butter or coconut oil) and reliance on fish as its primary source of animal protein to decrease the amount of saturated fats in the diet.

Other Conditions

As of 2022, the Mediterranean diet was ranked by *U.S. News & World Report* as the number one diet for overall health—for the fifth year in a row. Every year, a panel of twenty-five nationally recognized experts evaluate thirty-five of the most popular health-promoting diets. Evidenced-based with a long-standing history, the Mediterranean diet continues to receive national affirmation. Research shows promise that the Mediterranean diet, with its nutrient density and anti-inflammatory effects, may be helpful for those with asthma, cancer, Alzheimer's, and other chronic conditions, according to a 2019 article published in the *British Journal of Pharmacology*. Supportive factors include improved immunity, reduced systemic inflammation, reductions in free radical damage, protection against cell degeneration, and overall antioxidant support.

The Building Blocks of the Diet

The pesco-Mediterranean diet features a wide variety of healthy foods you can enjoy freely plus a smaller list of foods that you may enjoy in moderation. Once you understand how certain foods negatively impact heart health, you may want to avoid some foods completely.

Foods to Enjoy

Foods consumed in their whole form (whole foods), especially those from the plant kingdom, make up the backbone of the pesco-Mediterranean diet. These include fruits and veggies, oily fish and seafood, nuts and seeds, olives, beans, legumes, and whole grains.

VEGETABLES AND FRUIT

Dark leafy greens, such as spinach and kale, and broccoli, carrots, cauliflower, turnips, radishes, mushrooms, and eggplant are just some of the colorful vegetables included in the pesco-Mediterranean diet plan.

OILY FISH AND SEAFOOD

You may eat shrimp, salmon, scallops, trout, halibut, and snapper, just to name a few types of fish and seafood included in the diet. These foods provide macronutrient protein plus omega-3s. They also support your heart-healthy diet with vitamins and minerals including vitamins B_{12} and D, iron, copper, magnesium, and zinc.

NUTS AND SEEDS

Small handfuls of these crunchy "snack-worthy" morsels add healthy monounsaturated fats to your diet, which benefit your brain, skin, nails, and hair. Great choices include walnuts, almonds, hazelnuts, pumpkin seeds, flaxseed, and sunflower seeds.

BEANS, LEGUMES, AND WHOLE GRAINS

These filling foods provide heart-protective B-vitamins, plant-based protein, and dietary fiber. They'll help sustain your energy and keep you satisfied. Enjoy a variety, including lentils, black-eyed peas, black beans, cannellini beans, and chickpeas.

Foods to Enjoy in Moderation

Low-fat dairy and eggs are both satisfying proteins you may keep in your diet. They are even encouraged in the pesco-Mediterranean plan as long as you enjoy them in moderation. The same goes for wine and sweets, which, as we know, provide more for our soul's desire than our nutritional benefit.

DAIRY AND EGGS

Low-fat Greek yogurt is ideal for dishes like fruit parfaits, creamy salad dressings, and probiotic-rich dips. Use low-fat (1 percent) milk for enhancing creamy purees, adding to your coffee, or to whip up a batch of whole-grain pancakes. A variety of low-fat cheeses including mozzarella, feta, and goat cheese may be used to add flavor to leafy green salads and veggie-rich sandwiches. They can also be paired with veggies or fruit. Eggs are also a simple, convenient source of protein that can be prepared in a variety of delicious ways.

Note that low-fat dairy is advised because it is lower in saturated fats. However, a small dollop of cream or a sprinkling of (full-fat) feta may also be enjoyed as long as you keep it minimal. The good news is that a little can go a long way in flavoring a dish.

WINE

It's true that pressed grapes used to make wine add the benefit of resveratrol, an antioxidant known for its heart-protective properties, but enjoy this drink modestly. Alcohol can impair judgment, making it easier to abandon your healthy regime and consume more food than you need. It is also dehydrating. Enjoy alcohol with food, not on an empty stomach, and be sure to drink plenty of water.

SWEETS

Incorporate sweets minimally and only on occasion as they're packed with more sugars and starch than heart-healthy nutrients. Consider making your own treats with little to no added sugar. If you eat mindfully and slowly, you can enjoy each bite.

Foods to Minimize or Avoid

Certain foods and beverages may fill you up (temporarily) with little nutritional benefit. These foods are best to avoid and include refined grains, added sugars, highly processed foods, and foods that are high in sodium. This pesco-Mediterranean plan also discourages consumption of pork, chicken, and red meat to help minimize sodium and saturated fat in the diet.

REFINED GRAINS

Minimize your intake of breads, muffins, crackers, and pretzels. Ideally, you'll want to choose items that include at least 3 grams of fiber and less than 5 grams of sugar per serving. You may be surprised by how much sugar these foods contain despite the fact that they may not actually taste very sweet. And remember to always check the serving size.

ADDED SUGARS

Many highly processed packaged foods contain added sugars for flavor balance, sweetness, or preservation. These are items like energy and granola bars, sugary cereals, packaged muffins, cookies, pastries, and traditional sodas. Choose foods with 5 grams or less of added sugars per serving and stick to serving sizes indicated on the packaging. The American Heart Association recommends no more than 25 grams of added sugars per day for women and no more than 36 grams of added sugars per day for men.

HIGHLY PROCESSED FOODS

These include refined grains, added sugars, added sodium, and chemicals or additives that don't benefit our bodies. Many commercially packaged snack foods contain these ingredients and are designed for convenience, not nutrition.

HIGH-SODIUM FOODS

Highly processed foods account for much of the excess sodium in the typical American diet. Chips, pretzels, breads, and muffins have sodium levels that can add up over the course of a day. Also be mindful of traditional frozen food and options at restaurants, including meat lasagnas, fried chicken dishes, and meatloaf entrées. These may contain 1,000 milligrams of sodium—or more—per serving! It is also imperative you choose low-sodium canned foods.

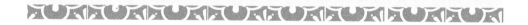

The Benefits of Intermittent Fasting

Intermittent fasting (IF) is a pattern in which you consume all your calories during a certain window of the day (e.g., eight hours) and fast during the remaining hours. While the fasting period is typically sixteen hours, some people choose to fast for twenty-four hours on alternate days or for two nonconsecutive days during the week.

IF is popular for weight loss and can be effective for limiting daily calories. It is proposed that caloric restriction improves insulin sensitivity and overall blood sugar levels, which is especially important for people with type 2 diabetes.

Science has also linked IF to improved gut health and disease prevention through cellular cleansing and renewal (autophagy), improvements in gut microbiome (fostering healthy bacteria), and anti-inflammatory benefits. Much of this research has been done on rats, not humans, yet it is still promising.

There may also be potential for IF's role in healing. A 2020 study in *Theranostics* found that "fasting with refeeding" accelerated wound healing in diabetic mice. The study suggests that IF proliferates new blood vessels that carry oxygen and nutrients to the wounded areas and influence collagen production to aid in healing and recovery.

You can safely incorporate IF into a pesco-Mediterranean dietary plan. Because IF is not a lengthy fast, it might be practical for some people. However, it is just one way of managing caloric intake. I do not recommend IF for someone with a history of disordered eating as it may increase the risk of binging or bulimic tendencies.

Serving Sizes for Common Foods

It is important to be mindful of your serving sizes so you can oversee the amount you eat. You don't want to leave your meal peckish, nor would you want to overstuff yourself. And it is a good way to ensure that you meet—not exceed—your calorie needs for the day.

A serving is a guideline for portioning out foods onto your plate (e.g., 4 ounces of fish or ¾ cup of potatoes). The serving guidelines in the visual chart that follows are based on caloric content (e.g., ¾ cup of pasta, rice, or potatoes is about 150 calories), although ½-cup servings are likely easier to calculate into a total day's needs. For adults on an 1,800- to 2,000-calorie diet, the current *Dietary Guidelines for Americans* suggest 2½ cups of vegetables per day. Five ½-cup servings will meet this goal.

	Equivalent	Food	Calories
	Fist (¾ cup)	Rice Pasta Potatoes	150 150 150
	Palm (4 ounces)	Lean meat Fish Poultry	160 160 160
	Handful (1 ounce)	Nuts Raisins	170 85
	Thumb (1 ounce)	Peanut butter Hard cheese	170 100

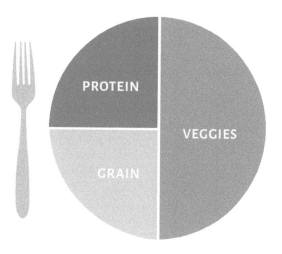

The Balanced Plate

You may be familiar with the approach of filling half your plate with veggies and fruit. This ensures that you get plenty of those nutrient-dense, antioxidant-rich foods in your diet. Fill the remainder of your plate with one-quarter protein and one-quarter whole grains or starchy vegetables.

And about that fat: Include it but don't go overboard; make wise choices. Fat helps support the flavors in your dish and improve the absorption of fat-soluble vitamins A, D, E, and K. Healthy fats include olives, olive oil, avocado, and a variety of nuts. You may also include some (mostly low-fat) cheese. There are so many delicious ways to pair healthy fats with your seafood, from Pistachio-Encrusted Scallops (page 108) to Mediterranean Snapper with Olives and Feta (page 113). And if you are enjoying a salad, a sprinkling of nuts and some avocado slices can add to its flavor and textural appeal.

Be mindful of your servings. Refer to Serving Sizes for Common Foods (page 12).

When it comes to packaged foods, be sure to read the labels. Often even a small package may include multiple servings. In general, stick mostly with whole foods like brown rice, oats, low-sodium canned beans, and lentils. The labels on the packages make it easy to identify a proper serving.

Making the Most of Your Healthy Diet

Staying on top of your health is more than just watching what you eat or drink; it also includes paying attention to how and when you eat and how you exercise and provide adequate rest for your brain and body. Finding a good lifestyle balance is essential for healthy, sustained energy levels and clarity of mind. Here are some key principles for a heart-healthy lifestyle.

Stay hydrated. Drink water throughout the day for its hydrating effect on your cells as well as its role in healthy blood circulation. Consuming water throughout the day keeps the heart pumping blood throughout the body and reduces strain on the muscles.

Plan your meals. Plan and prep a minimum of two or three dinners for the week, repurposing leftovers for the remainder of your afternoon and evening meals. Stick with simple, fuss-free breakfast combos using regularly stocked ingredients (e.g., a bowl of oatmeal with thawed frozen berries or all-natural peanut butter on whole grain toast). You may follow a specific meal plan like the four included in this book (see page 21). Shopping lists are included for your convenience.

Stock your kitchen wisely. Stock your kitchen with fresh and frozen veggies and fruit, canned beans, whole grains like oats and brown rice, olive oil, wild-caught tuna, and a variety of herbs and spices. It's a good idea to always have frozen options for veggies and fruits as fresh produce doesn't last very long. This way, even when you don't have a meal planned, you'll have plenty of options to build a healthy one.

Eat a variety of fruits and vegetables. Because every plant food has a specific amount, type, and range of essential nutrients, it's a good idea to enjoy a variety to ensure that you get adequate amounts of the nutrients you need. A variety also provides a wealth of flavor and texture options for your meals so you won't get bored eating the same things.

Practice mindful eating. Eat slowly, enjoy each bite, and focus on your meal (not your smartphone or the various tasks you have planned for the day). Studies show that taking the time to be in the moment increases your awareness of what and how much you are eating and better informs your satiety.

Incorporate daily exercise. Get your blood pumping and improve your circulation. Exercise is a great way to stay motivated and active both mentally and physically. It may also be a powerful mood booster and stress reliever. Alternate between weight training and cardio routines (and include some yoga) to meet your physical and mental needs.

What to Drink on the Mediterranean Diet

Water is the beverage of choice for a heart-healthy diet. You may also include tea and coffee in your daily ritual as well as wine, beer, and liquor on occasion.

According to the Mayo Clinic, men should aim to consume 15½ cups of water per day and women 11½ cups, but eight glasses of water per day for anyone is still a reasonable goal. Include green tea for its antioxidant benefits—it may be consumed throughout the day as its slow release of caffeine offers a steady energizing effect. Black tea may also be an option. Limit your coffee to one or two cups because the caffeine in coffee is known to cause jitters and even raise your blood pressure a bit, especially if you consume too much.

You may include alcohol on occasion. Alcohol not only lessens inhibitions, but it can also make you clumsier and less alert. Furthermore, these drinks don't provide much nutritional benefit for the body, even though wine is often touted for its antioxidant resveratrol, so sip a little at a time and enjoy. Recommended serving sizes are:

- 5 ounces of white or red wine
- 12 ounces of beer
- 1.5 ounces of hard liquor

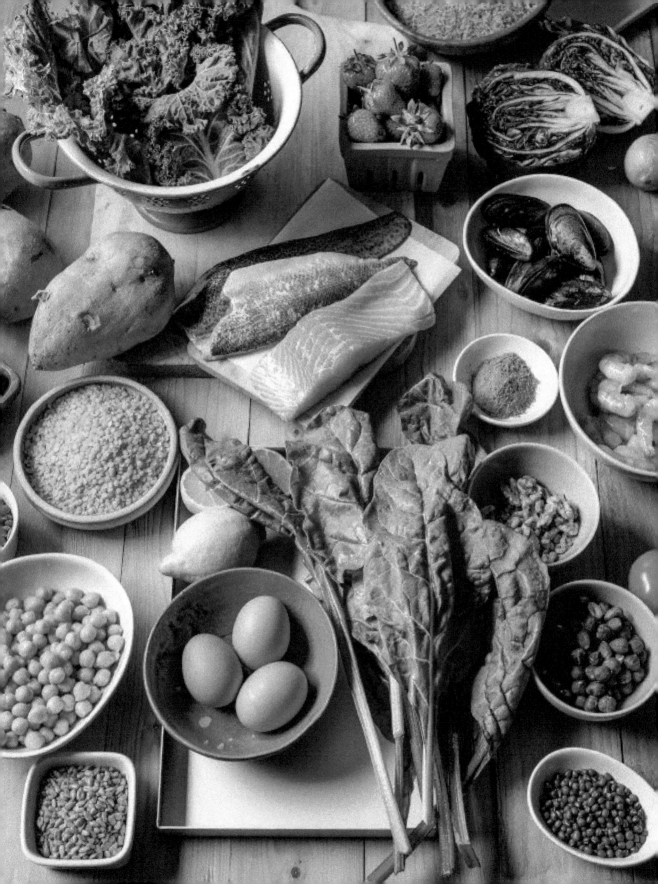

Chapter 2

The 28-Day Heart-Healthy Meal Plan

Ready to start improving your health? This chapter provides just what you need to start cooking the pesco-Mediterranean diet using fresh and quality whole food ingredients. Plus, you get four weeks of realistic and affordable meal plans.

Stocking Your Healthy Kitchen

To simplify your cooking, here are some ingredients you'll want to have on hand before you get started. Included are some recommended pantry staples for the refrigerator and freezer as well as some inexpensive, handy kitchen tools.

Refrigerator and Freezer Staples

You can count on some very common store-bought fresh and frozen ingredients for your dietary plan. These will serve as the backbone to several of the healthy pesco-Mediterranean diet recipes in this book.

- Carrots
- Cucumbers
- Eggs
- Fresh herbs (e.g., Italian parsley, basil, thyme, mint, rosemary, chives)
- Green beans (fresh or frozen)
- Jarred olives
- Leafy greens (e.g., kale, arugula, spinach, romaine lettuce)
- Mushrooms
- Salmon
- Shellfish (e.g., fresh or frozen shrimp, scallops)
- Whitefish (e.g., fresh or frozen halibut, tilapia, sole, cod)
- Zucchini

Pantry Staples

The recipes in this book lean heavily on some basic pantry items, most of which you likely already have. For those you don't have, you'll find acquiring some of these staples will serve you well.

- Balsamic vinegar
- Beans and legumes—if canned, look for low sodium; drain and rinse well before using (e.g., chickpeas, lentils, white beans)
- Canned fish (e.g., canned salmon, chunk albacore tuna)
- Canned tomatoes
- Dates
- Dried herbs and spices (coriander, oregano, cumin, nutmeg, black pepper, cinnamon, turmeric, salt, garlic powder, Italian seasoning)
- Extra-virgin olive oil
- Nuts and seeds
- Onions and garlic bulbs
- Rolled oats

Tools and Equipment

The recipes in this book use some of the most common kitchen tools and devices for cooking and storage.

- Baking dish
- Baking sheet
- Blender or food processor
- Dutch oven
- Large and medium stock pots
- Large and small skillets (oven-safe)

- Muffin tin

- Saucepans (large, medium, small)

- Set of mixing bowls, measuring cups, and measuring spoons

- Set of sharp knives

- Spatulas

- Stand mixer

- Tight-sealing storage containers (e.g., plastic zip-top bags, plastic or glass containers with lids, mason jars)

28 Days of Pesco-Mediterranean Diet Meals

When adjusting your diet, it's best to start simple. A no-fuss meal plan is a good way to get started. Each meal plan is designed with ten recipes per week to help you acclimate to a heart-healthy pesco-Mediterranean diet routine.

Each meal plan is designed for two people, but these plans can easily be scaled up or down. Most of the recipes in this book serve four, so intentional leftovers are built into each meal plan. If you are cooking for just yourself, I suggest you cut the recipes in half. Or you may choose to omit a couple of entrées, leveraging your leftovers to fill out the week. If you are feeding a family of four, double the recipes to have enough leftovers for those repeat meals intended for the week. Storage tips are provided at the end of each recipe.

Thinking of intermittent fasting? You will still be able to incorporate all the meals and snacks within each plan, you'll just be consuming them within a specific time window. Consider snacking only on a small piece of fruit or a handful of carrot sticks since your meals will be closer together with less time between.

Week 1 Meal Plan

	BREAKFAST	LUNCH	DINNER	SNACK
DAY 1	Loaded Avocado Sweet Potato "Toast" (page 42)	Citrus-Herb Scallops (page 98)	Greek Bean Soup (page 71)	¾ cup blueberries
DAY 2	*Leftover* Loaded Avocado Sweet Potato "Toast"	*Leftover* Greek Bean Soup	*Leftover* Citrus-Herb Scallops	Turmeric-Spiced Crispy Cauliflower (page 64)
DAY 3	Caprese Egg Muffin Cups (page 40)	Fresh Gazpacho Soup (page 81)	Lentil Burgers (page 74)	*Leftover* Turmeric-Spiced Crispy Cauliflower
DAY 4	*Leftover* Caprese Egg Muffin Cups	*Leftover* Fresh Gazpacho Soup	Tomatoes Stuffed with Herbed Bulgur (page 68)	4 ounces low-fat Greek yogurt + ½ cup berries
DAY 5	⅔ cup high-fiber, low-sugar cereal (e.g., Fiber One) + ½ cup almond milk	*Leftover* Tomatoes Stuffed with Herbed Bulgur	*Leftover* Lentil Burgers	¾ cup blueberries
DAY 6	⅔ cup high-fiber, low-sugar cereal (e.g., Fiber One) + ½ cup almond milk	*Leftover* Fresh Gazpacho Soup	Tuna Couscous Sauté (page 104)	Caramelized Sweet Potato Wedges (page 61)
DAY 7	1 cup of low-fat Greek yogurt + ½ cup berries	*Leftover* Tuna Couscous Sauté	*Leftover* Lentil Burgers	*Leftover* Caramelized Sweet Potato Wedges

Meal prep ahead of time: Caprese Egg Muffin Cups (page 40), Greek Bean Soup (page 71), Fresh Gazpacho Soup (page 81), Lentil Burgers (page 74)

The ingredients for this meal plan are easily accessible and can be found in most grocery stores. When shopping, look for the freshest options, although frozen vegetables (e.g., green beans) and fruits (e.g., berries) are also good choices. Since only one recipe in this plan calls for bread (and just two slices), feel free to choose a loaf of your choice—sourdough will substitute nicely for white, or use the pita (suggested in the recipe for the lentil burgers) instead. When tweaking a recipe to serve just one, you'll simply halve the recipes. To serve a family of four, double the recipes.

Week 1 Shopping List

PRODUCE

- ☐ Avocado, medium (1)
- ☐ Basil (1 large bunch)
- ☐ Carrots, large (4)
- ☐ Cauliflower (1 head)
- ☐ Celery (1 bunch)
- ☐ Cilantro (1 bunch)
- ☐ Cucumber, Persian (1)
- ☐ Garlic (1 bulb)
- ☐ Green beans (2 pounds)
- ☐ Italian parsley (1 bunch)

- ☐ Lemon (2)
- ☐ Lime (1)
- ☐ Mushrooms, cremini (8 ounces)
- ☐ Onion, yellow or white, large (1)
- ☐ Onion, sweet, large (1)
- ☐ Oregano, fresh (1 bunch)
- ☐ Potato, sweet, large (3)
- ☐ Thyme, fresh (1 bunch)
- ☐ Tomatoes, medium (2 pounds + 4)
- ☐ Zucchini, yellow (2)

DAIRY AND EGGS

- ☐ Eggs (1½ dozen)
- ☐ Greek yogurt, low-fat plain (32 ounces)

- ☐ Milk, 1 percent (1 pint)
- ☐ Mozzarella cheese, shredded, 1 (8-ounce) package

FRESH FISH AND SEAFOOD

☐ Scallops (1 pound)

FROZEN

☐ Blueberries 1 (32-ounce) package

HERBS AND SPICES

☐ Bay leaf

☐ Cayenne pepper, ground

☐ Cumin, ground

☐ Garlic powder

☐ Italian seasoning

☐ Paprika, smoked

☐ Red pepper flakes

☐ Turmeric, ground

PANTRY

☐ Albacore tuna, 2 (4-ounce) cans

☐ Almond milk, unsweetened, shelf stable (1 quart)

☐ Bread, sliced (1 loaf)

☐ Bulgur (1 cup)

☐ Cereal, low sugar (5 grams or less) and high fiber (3 grams or more), 1 standard box (e.g., Fiber One, Shredded Wheat, Cheerios)

☐ Couscous, 1 (6-ounce) package

☐ Flour, gluten-free, 1 (22-ounce) package

☐ Great northern beans, 1 (15-ounce) can

☐ Lentils, 1 (1-pound) bag

☐ Olive oil, extra-virgin

☐ Pita (1 package)

☐ Tomatoes, diced, 2 (15-ounce) cans

☐ Vinegar, red wine

OTHER

☐ White miso, 1 (14-ounce) package

Week 2 Meal Plan

	BREAKFAST	LUNCH	DINNER	SNACK
DAY 1	Greek Yogurt Parfait (page 50)	Freekeh Salad with Arugula and Peaches (page 70)	Quinoa and Goat Cheese–Stuffed Sweet Potato (page 88)—double the recipe	Fruit-Topped Meringues (page 127)
DAY 2	¼ cup granola + ¼ cup low-fat milk	*Leftover* Quinoa and Goat Cheese–Stuffed Sweet Potato	*Leftover* Freekeh Salad with Arugula and Peaches	Roasted Carrots with Spiced Yogurt and Granola (page 55)
DAY 3	*Leftover* Greek Yogurt Parfait	Mediterranean Salmon Wraps (page 110)—double the recipe	Mushroom and Potato Stew (page 86)	*Leftover* Fruit-Topped Meringues
DAY 4	Oatmeal (½ cup oats + water) + peach slices (1 peach)	*Leftover* Quinoa and Goat Cheese–Stuffed Sweet Potato	*Leftover* Mediterranean Salmon Wraps	*Leftover* Roasted Carrots with Spiced Yogurt and Granola
DAY 5	¼ cup granola + ¼ cup low-fat milk	*Leftover* Mediterranean Salmon Wraps	*Leftover* Mushroom and Potato Stew	1 cup sliced carrots
DAY 6	Oatmeal (½ cup oats + water) + peach slices (1 peach)	*Leftover* Mushroom and Potato Stew	Baked Spanish Salmon (page 106)	*Leftover* Roasted Carrots with Spiced Yogurt and Granola
DAY 7	¼ cup granola + ¼ cup low-fat milk	*Leftover* Baked Spanish Salmon	*Leftover* Quinoa and Goat Cheese–Stuffed Sweet Potato	*Leftover* Fruit-Topped Meringues

Meal prep ahead of time: Quinoa and Goat Cheese–Stuffed Sweet Potato (page 88), Mushroom and Potato Stew (page 86), Fruit-Topped Meringues (page 127)

Note: For the Greek Yogurt Parfait (page 50), assemble everything except the granola in advance to avoid soggy granola.

You should have no trouble finding these ingredients in most grocery stores. When grocery shopping, look for the freshest options available and do your best to streamline what you buy. For example, when it comes to tomatoes (e.g., Roma) buy or use any one type across the board as it may be easier or more cost effective. Freekeh, quinoa, and couscous may be used interchangeably, so buying one large package of one type of grain may be your preference. Cut the recipes in half to serve just one. Double the recipes to serve a family of four. *Note: The Quinoa and Goat Cheese–Stuffed Sweet Potato and Salmon Wraps are already doubled in this plan, so multiply the recipes by 4 if you have a family of four.*

Week 2 Shopping List

PRODUCE

☐ Arugula (5 ounces)

☐ Bell pepper, red, large (1)

☐ Carrots (2 bunches)

☐ Celery (1 bunch)

☐ Fennel bulb, large (1)

☐ Lemon (4)

☐ Mushrooms, white (5 ounces)

☐ Onion, red, small (3)

☐ Onion, yellow, small (1)

☐ Parsley (1 bunch)

☐ Peaches (6)

☐ Potato, russet (1)

☐ Potatoes, sweet (8)

☐ Romaine, large (1 head)

☐ Rosemary (15 sprigs)

☐ Tomatoes, cherry (1 cup)

☐ Tomato, Roma (3)

DAIRY AND EGGS

☐ Eggs (4)

☐ Feta cheese, crumbled (8 ounces)

☐ Goat cheese (8 ounces)

☐ Greek yogurt, low-fat plain (16 ounces + 8 ounces)

☐ Milk, low-fat (1 quart)

☐ Pecorino Romano (2 ounces)

FRESH FISH AND SEAFOOD

☐ Salmon, 4 (8-ounce) fillets

FROZEN

- ☐ Raspberries,
  1 (18-ounce) package

HERBS AND SPICES

- ☐ Bay leaf
- ☐ Cream of tartar
- ☐ Cumin seeds
- ☐ Garlic powder
- ☐ Paprika, smoked

PANTRY

- ☐ Almonds, slivered (2 ounces)
- ☐ Broth, low-sodium vegetable,
  1 (1-quart) container
- ☐ Chickpeas, 1 (15.5-ounce) can
- ☐ Couscous (1 cup)
- ☐ Freekeh (½ cup)
- ☐ Granola, 1 (8-ounce) package
- ☐ Honey
- ☐ Oats, rolled,
  1 (18-ounce) package
- ☐ Olives, Kalamata, 1 (8-ounce) jar
- ☐ Olives, pimento (15)
- ☐ Quinoa (1½ cups)
- ☐ Salmon, 4 (6-ounce) cans
- ☐ Tomatoes, diced, 1 (8-ounce) can
- ☐ Tortillas, whole wheat, 8 (6-inch)
- ☐ Vinegar, champagne

Week 3 Meal Plan

	BREAKFAST	LUNCH	DINNER	SNACK
DAY 1	6 ounces low-fat Greek yogurt + ½ cup blueberries	California Egg White Scramble (page 46)	Halibut with Shaved Fennel and Citrus Salad (page 102)	Spiced Oranges with Dates (page 122)
DAY 2	Apple Cinnamon Overnight Oats (page 44)—double the recipe	*Leftover* Halibut with Shaved Fennel and Citrus Salad	Lentil Ragout (page 90)	1 apple
DAY 3	*Leftover* Apple Cinnamon Overnight Oats	*Leftover* California Egg White Scramble	Shakshuka (page 48)	*Leftover* Spiced Oranges with Dates
DAY 4	Avocado-Blueberry Smoothie (page 47)	*Leftover* Lentil Ragout	Black-Eyed Peas and Kale Bowl (page 76)	½ avocado + lime juice + sea salt
DAY 5	6 ounces low-fat Greek yogurt + ½ cup blueberries	*Leftover* Shakshuka	*Leftover* Lentil Ragout	½ cup carrot sticks
DAY 6	Avocado-Blueberry Smoothie (page 47)	*Leftover* Black-Eyed Peas and Kale Bowl	Pistachio-Encrusted Scallops (page 108)	Coconut Date Energy Bites (page 126)
DAY 7	⅔ cup high-fiber, low-sugar cereal (e.g., Fiber One) + ½ cup 1 percent milk	*Leftover* Pistachio-Encrusted Scallops	*Leftover* Shakshuka	*Leftover* Coconut Date Energy Bites

Meal prep ahead of time: Lentil Ragout (page 90), Shakshuka (page 48), Coconut Date Energy Bites (page 126)

Note: Make the Avocado-Blueberry Smoothie (page 47) fresh each day.

You won't find it hard to locate the ingredients for the recipes in this plan because they are conveniently found in most major grocery outlets. While fresh and in-season produce provide optimal flavor and texture, frozen options of your favorite produce are also ideal for most dishes and are nutritious as well. Do your best to keep your shopping cart from overflowing by purchasing like items that are easily interchangeable. If you prefer plant-based milk, you may swap out the 1 percent milk for an equal amount of plant-based milk or vice versa. Choose just one type of milk for the week to save money and avoid waste. When tweaking a recipe for one serving, cut the recipe in half. To serve a family of four, double the recipes.

Week 3 Shopping List

PRODUCE

- Apples (3)
- Avocado, medium (4)
- Basil, fresh (1 small bunch)
- Bell pepper, green, large (1)
- Carrots, medium (1 bunch)
- Celery stalks (1 bunch)
- Chives (1 bunch)
- Cilantro (1 bunch)
- Fennel (2 bulbs)
- Garlic, large (1 bulb)
- Jalapeño (1)
- Kale (1 bunch)
- Lemon (1)
- Lime (2)
- Onion, sweet (1)
- Onion, yellow, medium (2)
- Oranges, blood (2)
- Oranges, medium (6)
- Parsley (1 bunch)
- Scallion (1 bunch)
- Shallot (1)
- Thyme, fresh (1 bunch)
- Tomatoes, cherry (1 cup)
- Tomatoes, large (2)

DAIRY AND EGGS

- Eggs (1½ dozen)
- Greek yogurt, low-fat plain (32 ounces + 8 ounces)
- Milk, 1 percent (1 quart)

FRESH FISH AND SEAFOOD

☐ Halibut, 4 (4-ounce) fillets

☐ Scallops (1 pound)

FROZEN

☐ Blueberries, 1 (32-ounce) package

HERBS AND SPICES

☐ Bay leaves

☐ Cayenne pepper

☐ Cinnamon, ground

☐ Cloves, ground

☐ Cumin, ground

☐ Oregano, dried

☐ Paprika, smoked

☐ Red pepper flakes

PANTRY

☐ Almond milk, unsweetened,
shelf-stable (1 quart)

☐ Black-eyed peas
2 (15-ounce) cans

☐ Broth, vegetable,
1 (1-quart) container

☐ Cereal, low sugar (5 grams or
less), high fiber (3 grams or more),
1 standard box (e.g., Fiber One,
Shredded Wheat, Cheerios)

☐ Chia seeds or flaxseed

☐ Coconut, unsweetened
shredded (½ cup)

☐ Dates, Medjool,
1 (16-ounce) package

☐ Hazelnuts, chopped,
1 (8-ounce) package

☐ Honey

☐ Lentils, French, green (1 pound)

☐ Maple syrup

☐ Oats, rolled 1 (18-ounce) package

☐ Oil, coconut

☐ Pistachios, unsalted (12 ounces)

☐ Rice, brown, 1 (8-ounce) package

☐ Tomatoes, whole peeled,
1 (28-ounce) can

☐ Vanilla extract

☐ Vinegar, red wine

☐ Vinegar, sherry

Week 4 Meal Plan

	BREAKFAST	LUNCH	DINNER	SNACK
DAY 1	Stuffed Cherry Tomatoes (page 62) + 1 scrambled egg	Crostini with Smoked Trout (page 41)—halve the recipe	Vegetable Paella (page 94)	*Leftover* from Week 3: Coconut Date Energy Bites
DAY 2	Tomato and Herb Baked Ricotta Toast (page 45)—only toast 2 slices of French baguette	*Leftover* Vegetable Paella	Mussels in Ginger-Garlic Broth (page 100)	*Leftover* Stuffed Cherry Tomatoes
DAY 3	*Leftover* Tomato and Herb Baked Ricotta Toast	*Leftover* Mussels in Ginger-Garlic Broth	*Leftover* Vegetable Paella	*Leftover* Stuffed Cherry Tomatoes
DAY 4	Hard-boiled egg (sliced) served with slices of ½ medium avocado (season with lemon and sea salt)	Crostini with Smoked Trout (page 41)—halve the recipe	Butternut Squash, Zucchini, and Bulgur Pilaf (page 95)	*Leftover* Coconut Date Energy Bites
DAY 5	*Leftover* Tomato and Herb Baked Ricotta Toast	*Leftover* Butternut Squash, Zucchini, and Bulgur Pilaf	Fiery Salmon Skewers (page 116)—double the recipe	*Leftover* Stuffed Cherry Tomatoes
DAY 6	Hard-boiled egg (sliced) served with ½ cup frozen (thawed) mixed berries	*Leftover* Fiery Salmon Skewers	Tomatoes Stuffed with Herbed Bulgur (page 68)	½ cup cucumber slices + 1 ounce crème fraîche
DAY 7	½ medium avocado + 1 scrambled egg	*Leftover* Tomatoes Stuffed with Herbed Bulgur	*Leftover* Fiery Salmon Skewers	½ cup cucumber slices + 1 ounce crème fraîche

Meal prep ahead of time: Vegetable Paella (page 94), Butternut Squash, Zucchini, and Bulgur Pilaf (page 95)

Note: For meals that require you to toast or grill the bread (e.g., Crostini with Smoked Trout and Tomato and Herb Baked Ricotta Toast), prepare only the amount you'll be eating. You can prepare/store everything else as directed.

For convenience and practicality, the ingredients for this plan are available in most major grocery stores. Fresh is always a good option, but frozen versions of fruit, veggies, or fish are just as nutritious. Thaw as necessary. To save time and money, you may opt for one type of a particular produce. For example, while specific recipes may call for sweet onions or yellow onions, you may swap one for the other as you prefer. Yellow and sweet onions are more easily interchangeable than red onions because they don't have the specific bite that red onions have. The baguette and sourdough loaf may also be used interchangeably. To tweak recipes for one serving, simply cut the recipes in half. To serve a family of four, double the recipes.

Week 4 Shopping List

PRODUCE

- ☐ Avocado (3)
- ☐ Basil (1 bunch)
- ☐ Bell pepper, green, large (1)
- ☐ Bell pepper, red, large (1)
- ☐ Butternut squash (3 pounds)
- ☐ Cilantro (1 bunch)
- ☐ Cucumber, medium (1)
- ☐ Dill (1 small packet)
- ☐ Garlic (2 large bulbs)
- ☐ Ginger root (1)
- ☐ Jalapeño (1)
- ☐ Lemon (1)
- ☐ Lemon, Meyer (1)
- ☐ Lime (2)
- ☐ Onion, red, large (2)
- ☐ Onion, sweet, large (2)
- ☐ Onion, yellow, small (1)
- ☐ Oregano, fresh (1 packet)
- ☐ Parsley (1 bunch)
- ☐ Rosemary (1 small packet)
- ☐ Scallions (1 bunch)
- ☐ Tomatoes, cherry (2 pints)
- ☐ Tomatoes, large (10)
- ☐ Zucchini, medium (2)

DAIRY AND EGGS

☐ Crème fraîche,
   1 (8-ounce) container

☐ Eggs, medium (1 dozen)

☐ Ricotta cheese, part-skim,
   1 (16-ounce) container

FRESH FISH AND SEAFOOD

☐ Mussels, fresh (1½ pounds)

☐ Salmon, skinless (1 pound)

FROZEN

☐ Green beans (16 ounces)

☐ Mixed berries,
   1 (16-ounce) package

HERBS AND SPICES

☐ Cayenne pepper

☐ Cumin, ground

☐ Italian seasoning

☐ Onion powder

☐ Paprika, smoked

☐ Saffron threads (optional)

☐ Turmeric

PANTRY

☐ Bread, sourdough (1 loaf)

☐ Broth, vegetable,
   1 (1-quart) container

☐ Bulgur (1½ cups)

☐ French baguette (1)

☐ Rice, short-grain (1½ cups)

☐ Smoked trout, 1 (4-ounce) can

☐ Vinegar, red wine

☐ Walnuts (¼ cup)

☐ Wine, white (Chardonnay works
   well), 1 bottle

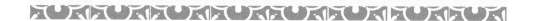

Eating After 28 Days

Once you've completed your 28 days, you may be wondering what to eat. Building your own weekly meal plan can be a cinch with a few simple strategies.

Overall, you need to plan for only six meals—that's six dinners with leftovers eaten for lunch the next day. Dinner on day 7 can be healthy takeout or a quick combo of ingredients you have on hand. (In a pinch, you can throw together a stir-fry with broccoli, bell pepper, onions, and tofu or build an omelet with many of the same ingredients.) To get started, choose one fish dish and one vegetarian entrée; then list all the ingredients on a sheet of paper. Build four additional entrée combos by pairing protein and veggies inspired by ingredients on your list. Consider your carbs: Will the entrée be served with rice, potato, or beans? These are ingredients you likely already have in your cupboard. Just because something like fish-taco filling is typically served in a tortilla, it doesn't mean you have to eat it that way. Be sure to calculate for extra produce, fish, or other ingredients you'll need for those additional meals.

Breakfast can be as simple as cereal and milk or a scrambled egg on whole grain toast. (For a quick and easy nutritional boost, add fresh berries to your cereal and spinach to your scramble.) Ideally you'll be using items you typically have on hand or from a bulk ingredient included in one of the recipes (e.g., eggs are usually bought by the dozen). Snacks can be a piece of fresh fruit and/or a loose handful of nuts.

If you'd prefer more flexibility than a detailed meal plan provides, be sure to have three or four protein options (e.g., eggs, tofu, salmon, beans) and a variety of veggies you can mix and match.

The Recipes in This Book

As you scan through the pesco-Mediterranean diet recipes in this book, keep in mind that these dishes can be enjoyed à la carte or as part of a complete entrée. You can even turn an appetizer into a meal by adding your choice of protein. For example, prepare the Stuffed Cherry Tomatoes (page 62) and serve the dish with 4 ounces of grilled salmon. Fish dishes like Pan-Seared Shrimp Skewers (page 109) can be made more satisfying with a side of quinoa or wild rice to add some dietary fiber and a side of steamed broccoli.

These recipes were created with your convenience and preference in mind. Dietary labels of "Vegetarian" and "Dairy-Free" make it easy to spot recipes that fit your needs. Convenience labels include "Quick" (less than 30 minutes from start to finish) and "1-Pot Meal" (uses just one cooking pot or pan to cook an entrée). Some recipes are made with and labeled "5 or Fewer Ingredients" (not counting common pantry staples like salt, pepper, olive oil, and nonstick cooking spray), and some recipes may take more than 45 minutes to prepare from start to finish and are labeled "Worth the Wait."

With substitution tips, variation options, shopping tips, and nutritional information, you have what you need to follow a healthy eating plan with practicality and convenience in mind. You'll have plenty of flavorful dishes to enjoy as well as inspiration for many more healthy meals to come.

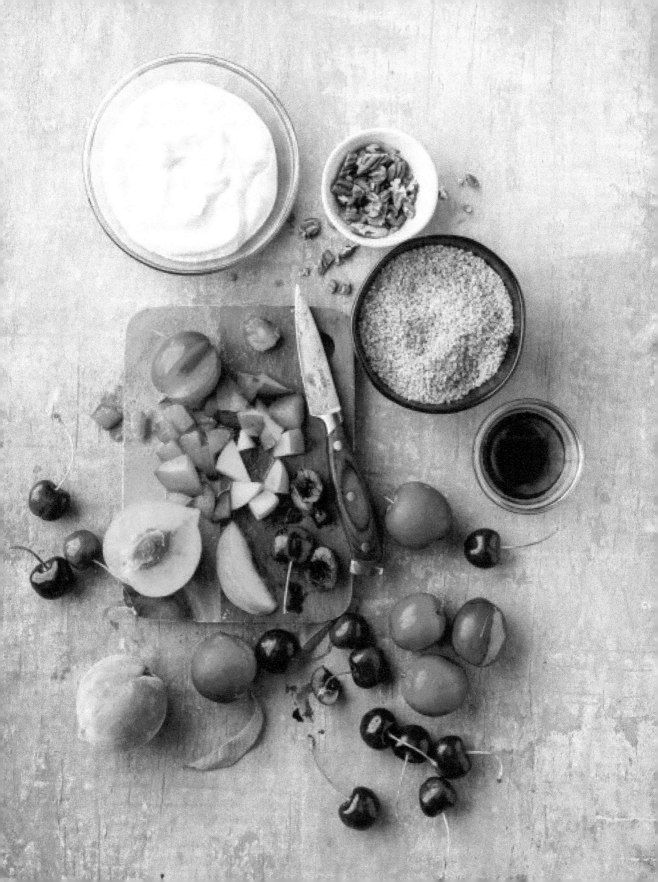

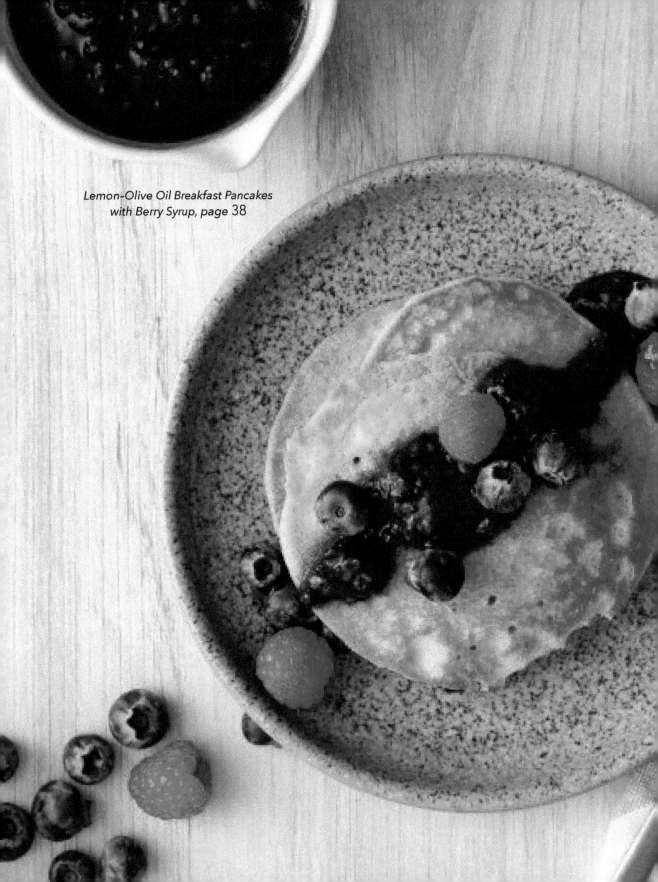

*Lemon–Olive Oil Breakfast Pancakes
with Berry Syrup, page 38*

Chapter 3

Breakfast

Lemon–Olive Oil Breakfast Pancakes with Berry Syrup

DAIRY-FREE
VEGETARIAN
QUICK

Serves 4
Prep time: 5 minutes / Cook time: 20 minutes

Weekends are made for pancakes! Olive oil–based pancakes are a common staple for the Mediterranean baker. The lemon flavor in these breakfast pancakes is a light and refreshing new twist on a breakfast favorite. And with berries in the mix, you get immune-boosting antioxidants. Garnish with fresh berries as desired.

FOR THE PANCAKES

1 cup almond flour
1 teaspoon baking powder
¼ teaspoon salt
6 tablespoons extra-virgin olive oil, divided
2 large eggs
Grated zest and juice of 1 lemon
½ teaspoon almond or vanilla extract

FOR THE BERRY SYRUP

1 cup frozen mixed berries
1 tablespoon water or lemon juice, plus more if needed
½ teaspoon vanilla extract

TO MAKE THE PANCAKES

1. In a large bowl, combine the almond flour, baking powder, and salt and whisk to break up any clumps.

2. Add 4 tablespoons of olive oil, the eggs, grated lemon zest and juice, and almond extract and whisk to combine well.

3. In a large skillet, heat 1 tablespoon of olive oil over medium heat and spoon about 2 tablespoons of batter for each of the 4 pancakes into the skillet. Cook until bubbles begin to form, 4 to 5 minutes, and flip. Cook 2 to 3 minutes more on the second side. Repeat with the remaining 1 tablespoon of olive oil and the remaining batter.

4. Leftover pancakes can be frozen in an airtight container for up to 2 months.

TO MAKE THE BERRY SYRUP

5. In a small saucepan, heat the frozen berries, water, and vanilla over medium-high heat for 3 to 4 minutes, until bubbly, adding more water if the mixture is too thick. Using the back of a spoon or fork, mash the berries, and whisk until smooth.

6. Refrigerate in an airtight container for 2 to 3 days.

PREP TIP: To save money, you can make your own almond flour by processing raw (or blanched) almonds in your food processor. Add 1 cup of almonds to your food processor with the blade attachment, and pulse repeatedly for about 1 minute until all bits are ground to a flour consistency.

Per serving (2 pancakes with ¼ cup berry syrup): Calories: 379; Total Fat: 35g; Saturated Fat: 5g; Cholesterol: 93mg; Sodium: 273mg; Potassium: 248mg; Magnesium: 71mg; Carbohydrates: 12g; Sugars: 5g; Fiber: 4g; Protein: 8g; Added Sugars: 0g; Vitamin K: 19mcg

Caprese Egg Muffin Cups

Serves 4
Prep time: 10 minutes / Cook time: 25 minutes

Whether you are on the go or busy at home, these protein-rich caprese egg muffins will simplify your morning breakfast routine. There are some egg whites in the mix to keep the egg muffins lower in saturated fats yet still fluffy and satisfying. Make a batch to last your entire week.

6 large eggs
4 egg whites
½ cup 1 percent milk
⅛ teaspoon salt
Freshly ground black pepper
2 teaspoons Italian seasoning
1 cup diced tomatoes
⅓ cup shredded mozzarella cheese
½ cup roughly chopped fresh basil, lightly packed
Nonstick cooking spray

1. Preheat the oven to 350°F.

2. Whisk together the eggs, egg whites, and milk in a bowl. Season with salt, pepper, and Italian seasoning. Add the tomatoes, mozzarella cheese, and basil to the bowl. Stir until everything is well combined.

3. Coat a 12-cup muffin tin with cooking spray. Fill the muffin cups halfway with the egg mixture.

4. Bake for 20 to 25 minutes, until the centers are set and no longer runny. Allow to cool slightly before serving.

5. Refrigerate in an airtight container for up to 5 days and reheat in the microwave before serving.

PREP TIP: These egg muffins are freezer-friendly, too! Make an extra batch, let cool, and wrap each muffin individually in aluminum foil. When you're looking for a quick breakfast, remove foil and defrost in the microwave before rushing out the door.

Per serving (3 muffins): Calories: 174; Total Fat: 10g; Saturated Fat: 4g; Cholesterol: 288mg; Sodium: 313mg; Potassium: 326mg; Magnesium: 25mg; Carbohydrates: 4g; Sugars: 3g; Fiber: 1g; Protein: 16g; Added Sugars: 0g; Vitamin K: 17mcg

Crostini with Smoked Trout

1 POT MEAL
QUICK

Serves 4
Prep time: 10 minutes / Cook time: 5 minutes
5 or Fewer Ingredients

Trout is a good source of omega-3s, protein, and vitamin D, and the smoked version of trout is tasty and ready to eat. This version is served on a baguette toasted with olive oil and seasoning and topped with crème fraîche and fresh dill for a refreshing flavor. It is perfect for a crowd-pleasing hors d'oeuvre. To make it a meal, just double your portion and serve it with some leafy greens.

½ French baguette, cut into 1-inch-thick slices
1 tablespoon extra-virgin olive oil
¼ teaspoon onion powder
1 (4-ounce) can smoked trout
¼ cup crème fraîche
¼ teaspoon chopped fresh dill, for garnish

1. Drizzle the bread on both sides with the olive oil and sprinkle with the onion powder.

2. Place the bread in a single layer in a large skillet and toast over medium heat until lightly browned on both sides, 3 to 4 minutes total.

3. Transfer the toasted bread to a serving platter and place one or two pieces of the trout on each slice. Top with the crème fraîche, garnish with the dill, and serve immediately.

4. Store leftovers at room temperature in an airtight container for 5 to 7 days. If you are making these in advance, it is best to add the crème fraîche and fresh dill just before serving.

PREP TIP: Instead of toasting the bread in a skillet, you can arrange the slices on a baking sheet and toast them under the broiler in a preheated oven until lightly browned on both sides, about 30 seconds per side.

Per serving: Calories: 265; Total Fat: 8g; Saturated Fat: 2g; Cholesterol: 32mg; Sodium: 467mg; Potassium: 283mg; Magnesium: 33mg; Carbohydrates: 30g; Sugars: 3g; Fiber: 1g; Protein: 17g; Added Sugars: 0g; Vitamin K: 3mcg

Loaded Avocado Sweet Potato "Toast"

Serves 4
Prep time: 5 minutes / Cook time: 15 minutes
5 or Fewer Ingredients

If you are watching your carbs, this avocado "toast" is ideal for you—there are only 11 grams of carbohydrates per serving. Sweet potato offers plenty of fiber, beta-carotene, and B-vitamins. And the creamy avocado is a good source of fiber, too. Healthy fats and fiber make this quick and easy breakfast (or snack option) ideal for controlling appetite and blood sugar.

1 avocado, pitted and peeled
Salt
Freshly ground black pepper
1 large sweet potato, scrubbed with skin on and cut lengthwise into 4 slices
4 eggs
1 teaspoon fresh thyme, for garnish

1. Preheat oven to 375°F.

2. In a small bowl, mash the avocado and season with salt and black pepper. Set aside.

3. Place the sweet potato slices on a baking sheet lined with aluminum foil or parchment paper. Bake for 15 to 20 minutes, turning once halfway through. Bake until the sweet potato gets soft, slightly caramelized, and crispy along the edge.

4. Prepare the eggs whichever way you desire: hard-boiled, scrambled, poached, over easy, or sunny-side up.

5. Transfer each sweet potato slice to a plate. Top each slice with a quarter of the mashed avocado and an egg. Sprinkle with salt, black pepper, thyme, and red pepper flakes.

6. Refrigerate the leftovers in an airtight container for 3 to 5 days.

Per serving: Calories: 180; Total Fat: 12g; Saturated Fat: 3g; Cholesterol: 186mg; Sodium: 131mg; Potassium: 423mg; Magnesium: 29mg; Carbohydrates: 11g; Sugars: 2g; Fiber: 4g; Protein: 8g; Added Sugars: 0g; Vitamin K: 11mcg

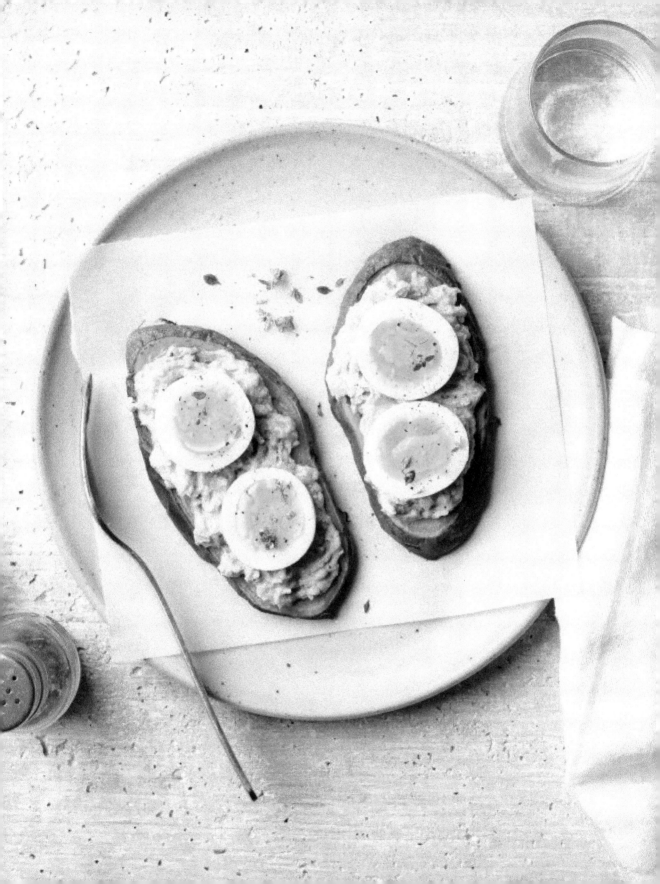

Apple Cinnamon Overnight Oats

Serves 2
Prep time: 15 minutes, plus at least 4 hours refrigeration

This breakfast is a mash-up of sweet morning oatmeal and freshly baked apple pie. Besides the classic flavor combination of apples and cinnamon, the best part about these overnight oats is that they're quick to make, use ingredients most of us have on hand, and are prepared ahead, making weekday mornings stress-free and delicious.

1 cup old-fashioned rolled oats
2 tablespoons chia seeds or ground flaxseed
1¼ cups 1 percent milk
½ tablespoon ground cinnamon
2 teaspoons honey or pure maple syrup
½ teaspoon vanilla extract
Dash salt
1 apple, diced

1. Divide the oats, chia seeds, milk, cinnamon, honey, vanilla, and salt into two mason jars. Place the lids tightly on top and shake until thoroughly combined.

2. Remove the lids and add half of the diced apple to each jar. Sprinkle with additional cinnamon, if desired. Place the lids tightly on the jars and refrigerate for at least 4 hours or overnight.

3. Refrigerate in single-serve airtight containers for up to 3 days.

PREP TIP: Any milk (cow's, almond, soy, coconut) can be used in this recipe.

STORAGE TIP: If you don't have mason jars, simply whisk the overnight oat mixture in a bowl and transfer it to containers with airtight lids.

SUBSTITUTION TIP: Replace the cinnamon and apples with mango and coconut for tropical overnight oats.

Per serving: Calories: 392; Total Fat: 9g; Saturated Fat: 2g; Cholesterol: 8mg; Sodium: 149mg; Potassium: 598mg; Magnesium: 153mg; Carbohydrates: 65g; Sugars: 17g; Fiber: 13g; Protein: 16g; Added Sugars: 6g; Vitamin K: 3mcg

Tomato and Herb Baked Ricotta Toast

VEGETARIAN
QUICK

Serves 6
Prep time: 5 minutes / Cook time: 15 minutes

The combination of herbs in this recipe's ricotta makes for a unique, fragrant piece of delicious toast. Parsley is a good source of essential vitamins A, C, and K. Basil supports eye health, and rosemary and oregano add antibacterial properties to the mix. Enjoy this dish for breakfast, as a snack, or as a crowd-pleasing appetizer—it's ideal for just about any occasion.

2 tablespoons extra-virgin olive oil, divided
1 tablespoon red wine vinegar
1 garlic clove, minced
1 pint cherry tomatoes, halved
Salt
Freshly ground black pepper
1 (8-ounce) container part-skim ricotta cheese
¼ cup coarsely chopped fresh basil
¼ cup coarsely chopped fresh parsley
2 tablespoons finely chopped fresh oregano
1 tablespoon finely chopped fresh rosemary
6 (¾-inch-thick) slices sourdough bread

1. Preheat the oven to 400°F.

2. In a medium bowl, whisk together 1 tablespoon of oil and the red wine vinegar. Add the garlic and cherry tomatoes, and season with salt and pepper. Mix until combined and set aside.

3. In another medium bowl, combine the ricotta, basil, parsley, oregano, and rosemary.

4. Line up the sourdough slices on a baking sheet. Brush each side of the bread with the remaining 1 tablespoon of olive oil. Scoop some of the herbed ricotta on top of each slice of bread. Top with the tomato mixture, pressing down so the tomatoes sink into the ricotta. Bake for 10 to 15 minutes, or until the tomatoes begin to blister and the cheese is golden.

5. You can prepare this in advance and refrigerate the tomato mixture and cheese blend in separate airtight containers for up to 7 days.

PREP TIP: If prepping in advance, make the toast and assemble it on the day you plan to serve the dish.

Per serving: Calories: 186; Total Fat: 8g; Saturated Fat: 3g; Cholesterol: 12mg; Sodium: 259mg; Potassium: 165mg; Magnesium: 21mg; Carbohydrates: 20g; Sugars: 2g; Fiber: 1g; Protein: 8g; Added Sugars: 0g; Vitamin K: 50mcg

California Egg White Scramble

Serves 4
Prep time: 20 minutes / Cook time: 5 minutes

Don't let this recipe's name fool you. Its ingredients—fresh herbs, extra-virgin olive oil, avocado, and tomatoes—are popular in the Mediterranean as well as in California for their high nutritional impact. Thyme supports a healthy digestive system, relieves respiratory conditions and arthritis, and detoxifies the liver.

10 large egg whites
1 tablespoon chopped fresh parsley
1 teaspoon chopped fresh basil
½ teaspoon chopped fresh thyme
Salt
Freshly ground black pepper
1 tablespoon extra-virgin olive oil
1 ripe avocado, pitted, peeled, and chopped
1 cup halved cherry tomatoes, at room temperature
1 scallion, both white and green parts, thinly sliced on the bias
2 tablespoons chopped fresh cilantro
1 tablespoon minced jalapeño

1. In a medium bowl, whisk together the egg whites, parsley, basil, and thyme and season with salt and pepper.

2. In a large skillet, heat the olive oil over medium heat. Pour the egg mixture into the skillet and swirl the pan lightly. Scramble the eggs until cooked through but still moist, about 5 minutes.

3. Spoon the eggs onto a platter and top with the avocado, tomatoes, scallion, cilantro, and jalapeño. Serve.

4. Refrigerate the leftovers in an airtight container for 3 to 4 days.

SUBSTITUTION TIP: If you are using dried herbs instead of fresh, use a third the amount of the fresh herbs called for in the recipe. Thus, you would swap 1 tablespoon of fresh parsley for 1 teaspoon of dried parsley. For amounts too small to divide (such as ½ teaspoon), use just a pinch of the herb.

Per serving: Calories: 162; Total Fat: 11g; Saturated Fat: 2g; Cholesterol: 0mg; Sodium: 183mg; Potassium: 490mg; Magnesium: 31mg; Carbohydrates: 7g; Sugars: 2g; Fiber: 4g; Protein: 10g; Added Sugars: 0g; Vitamin K: 43mcg

Avocado-Blueberry Smoothie

Serves 2
Prep time: 5 minutes

Some smoothies are snacks or a light breakfast, but you will be satisfied and full of energy with this combination of yogurt, avocado, oats, and sweet blueberries. Blueberries are ranked at the top of the list of produce for antioxidant capabilities. They are absolutely packed with phytonutrients, anti-inflammatories, calcium, iron, folic acid, and B-vitamins. Enjoy blueberries several times a week to cut your risk of cancer, diabetes, bladder issues, heart disease, and cognitive diseases. Blueberries also help stabilize blood sugar and promote good eye health.

½ cup unsweetened almond milk

½ cup low-fat plain Greek yogurt

1 ripe avocado, peeled, pitted, and coarsely chopped

1 cup blueberries

¼ cup gluten-free rolled oats

½ teaspoon vanilla extract

4 ice cubes

1. In a blender, combine the almond milk, yogurt, avocado, blueberries, oats, and vanilla and pulse until well blended.

2. Add the ice cubes and blend until thick and smooth. Serve.

3. While smoothies are best served fresh, you can refrigerate the mixture in an airtight container for up to 1 day. Be sure to choose a container that the smoothie will fill to the brim to prevent oxidation.

SUBSTITUTION TIP: The yogurt can be omitted for vegans or people with dairy allergies. Try a couple tablespoons of coconut cream instead or a soy or coconut yogurt for extra creaminess.

Per serving: Calories: 328; Total Fat: 18g; Saturated Fat: 3g; Cholesterol: 4mg; Sodium: 89mg; Potassium:786 mg; Magnesium: 76mg; Carbohydrates: 38g; Sugars: 16g; Fiber: 10g; Protein: 9g; Added Sugars: 0g; Vitamin K: 36mcg

Shakshuka

Serves 6
Prep time: 10 minutes / Cook time: 30 minutes

Shakshuka originated in Tunisia but has become a popular breakfast dish across the Mediterranean region. Eggs are poached in a chunky, spicy tomato sauce along with sweet peppers, onions, and garlic for a savory dish you won't soon forget. Serve it with crusty bread.

¼ cup extra-virgin olive oil
1 onion, chopped
1 green bell pepper, seeded and chopped
1 garlic clove, minced
1 teaspoon smoked paprika
½ teaspoon ground cumin
¼ teaspoon red pepper flakes
Pinch salt
Freshly ground black pepper
1 (28-ounce) can whole peeled tomatoes
6 large eggs
¼ cup chopped fresh flat-leaf parsley

1. In a large skillet, heat the olive oil over medium heat. Cook the onion, bell pepper, garlic, paprika, cumin, red pepper flakes, salt, and black pepper for about 10 minutes, stirring often, until the vegetables soften.

2. Add the tomatoes with their juices and break apart with a potato masher or spoon. Cook the mixture for 10 minutes.

3. Using a spoon, make six wells in the mixture. Crack an egg into each well.

4. Cover the pan, reduce the heat to low, and simmer for 8 to 10 minutes, until the egg whites set and the yolks are still runny.

5. Garnish with chopped parsley.

6. Refrigerate the leftovers in an airtight container for 5 to 7 days. (The spices will meld and you'll get an even more intense flavor.) It's best to reheat on the stove (not in the microwave) to keep the eggs from getting rubbery.

Per serving: Calories: 187; Total Fat: 14g; Saturated Fat: 3g; Cholesterol: 186mg; Sodium: 253mg; Potassium: 411mg; Magnesium: 26mg; Carbohydrates: 8g; Sugars: 5g; Fiber: 3g; Protein: 8g; Added Sugars: 0g; Vitamin K: 52mcg

PREP TIP: To make this dish even spicier, sprinkle red pepper flakes on top just before serving. You can also serve this with a dollop of plain yogurt on top.

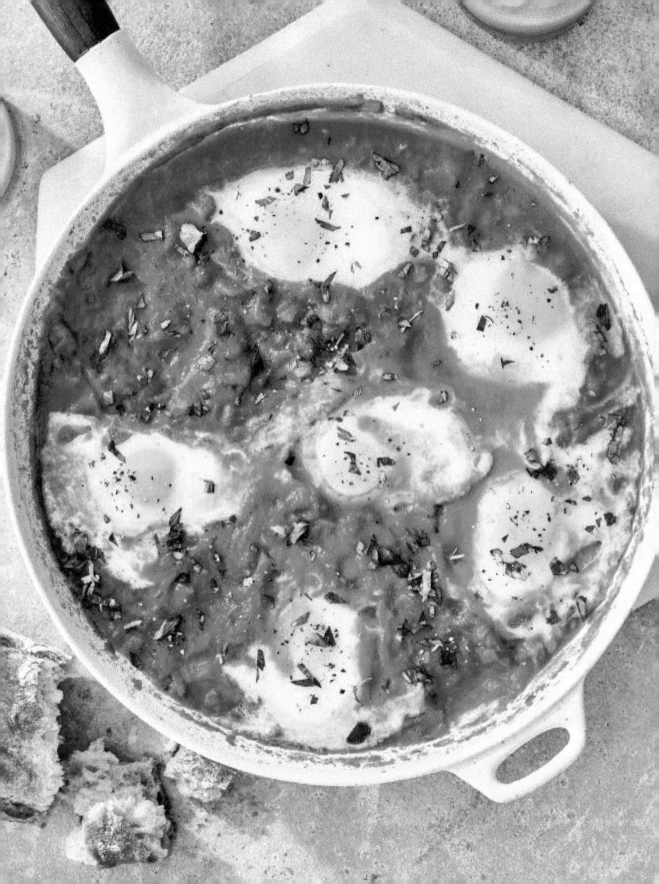

Greek Yogurt Parfait

Serves 4
Prep time: 10 minutes
5 or Fewer Ingredients

A classic Greek yogurt parfait is a decadent yet balanced breakfast that is super easy to make. Greek yogurt is a great source of protein, calcium, and probiotics, which support digestive health. It's thicker and creamier than regular yogurt.

2 cups low-fat plain Greek yogurt, divided
1 cup chopped raspberries, divided
1 cup granola
¼ cup chopped almonds
¼ cup honey

Spoon ¼ cup of yogurt into each of four wine glasses or mason jars. Arrange a layer of berries on top; then add ¼ cup more of yogurt. Top with the remaining berries, the granola, and almonds. Drizzle with the honey.

PREP TIP: To make vanilla yogurt, stir 1 teaspoon of vanilla into 2 cups of yogurt.

STORAGE TIP: You can prepare these parfaits up to 2 days in advance without the granola. Refrigerate in an airtight container for 2 or 3 days; then add the granola just before serving.

Per serving: Calories: 273; Total Fat: 7g; Saturated Fat: 2g; Cholesterol: 7mg; Sodium: 88mg; Potassium: 467mg; Magnesium: 74mg; Carbohydrates: 44g; Sugars: 11g; Fiber: 5g; Protein: 11g; Added Sugars: 17g; Vitamin K: 3mcg

Fresh Fruit Crumble Muesli

Serves 4
Prep time: 20 minutes

You might think you are eating dessert for breakfast when you take your first luscious bite of the sweet fruit and rich, nutty topping in this recipe. You can change the mixture of fruit to anything you happen to have on hand. The pecans in the topping can help reduce inflammation in the body, support a healthy cardiovascular system, and improve brain function.

1 cup gluten-free
 rolled oats
¼ cup chopped pecans
¼ cup almonds
4 pitted Medjool dates
1 teaspoon vanilla
 extract
¼ teaspoon ground
 cinnamon
1 cup sliced fresh
 strawberries
1 nectarine, pitted and
 chopped
2 kiwi, peeled and
 chopped
½ cup blueberries
1 cup low-fat plain
 Greek yogurt

1. In a food processor, combine the oats, pecans, almonds, dates, vanilla, and cinnamon and pulse until the mixture resembles coarse crumbs.

2. In a medium bowl, stir together the strawberries, nectarine, kiwi, and blueberries until well mixed. Divide the fruit and yogurt among four bowls and top each bowl with the oat mixture. Serve.

3. Refrigerate in single-serve airtight containers for up to 2 days.

PREP TIP: Many grocery stores carry date paste in the baking section, which is less expensive than whole dates. If you are pureeing or blending the fruit with other ingredients, as in this recipe, date paste is a great alternative.

Per serving: Calories: 331; Total Fat: 11g; Saturated Fat: 2g; Cholesterol: 4mg; Sodium: 45mg; Potassium: 668mg; Magnesium: 103mg; Carbohydrates: 51g; Sugars: 28g; Fiber: 8g; Protein: 11g; Added Sugars: 0g; Vitamin K: 6mcg

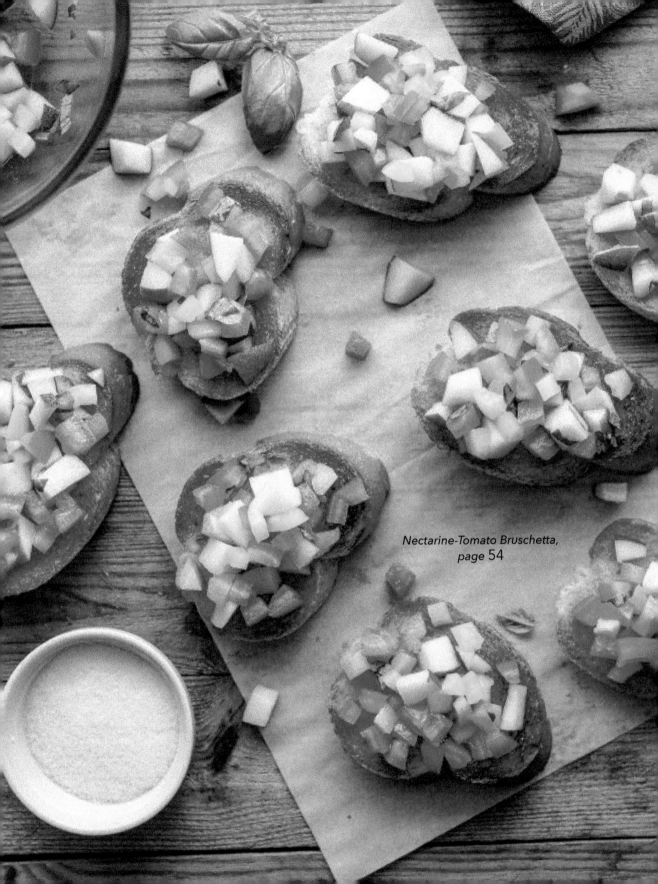

Nectarine-Tomato Bruschetta,
page 54

Chapter 4

Sides and Snacks

Nectarine-Tomato Bruschetta

Serves 4
Prep time: 15 minutes / Cook time: 5 minutes

Bruschetta is a stunning dish that is simple to create but looks like it took you hours. The most important aspect of bruschetta is the lightly grilled or broiled bread brushed with olive oil—so do not skip this step. The nectarine-tomato topping is sweet and tart and so beautiful that you might end up gazing at it for a minute before digging in.

2 nectarines, pitted and roughly chopped
1 large tomato, seeded and finely chopped
½ yellow bell pepper, seeded and finely chopped
1 tablespoon finely chopped fresh basil
Salt
Freshly ground black pepper
1 French baguette, cut into 8 (½-inch-thick) slices
1 tablespoon extra-virgin olive oil

1. Preheat the oven to broil.

2. In a medium bowl, stir together the nectarines, tomato, bell pepper, and basil. Season the bruschetta mixture with salt and pepper.

3. Place the bread slices on a baking sheet and brush lightly with olive oil.

4. Broil the bread until crispy and lightly golden, about 1 minute.

5. Use a slotted spoon to evenly divide the bruschetta mixture onto the broiled bread and serve immediately.

6. Refrigerate the nectarine and tomato mixture for up to 3 days. It is best to prepare the toast and assemble it on the day you plan to serve the dish.

Per serving: Calories: 261; Total Fat: 5g; Saturated Fat: 1g; Cholesterol: 0mg; Sodium: 459mg; Potassium: 383mg; Magnesium: 33mg; Carbohydrates: 47g; Sugars: 9g; Fiber: 4g; Protein: 9g; Added Sugars: 0g; Vitamin K: 10mcg.

PREP TIP: If you enjoy a little heat in your food, adding hot peppers to this recipe produces excellent results. Add 1 teaspoon of chopped hot pepper to the other ingredients in step 2. Jalapeño will provide a milder sensation, whereas a habanero or serrano pepper will have a much stronger kick.

Roasted Carrots with Spiced Yogurt and Granola

VEGETARIAN

Serves 4 to 6
Prep time: 10 minutes / Cook time: 30 minutes

Sweet roasted carrots paired with creamy yogurt and crunchy granola is as unique as it is nutritious. Carrots are rich in beta-carotene, an antioxidant that supports eye health and immunity. Yogurt offers probiotic benefits for healthy digestion. And crunchy granola provides fiber and heart-healthy B-vitamins. This may not be a combo you are familiar with, but after trying one bite, you will be hooked!

1 bunch tricolored
  carrots, trimmed and
  peeled
1 tablespoon
  extra-virgin olive oil
2 tablespoons honey,
  divided
Kosher salt
Freshly ground black
  pepper
½ cup low-fat plain
  Greek yogurt
2 teaspoons finely
  chopped fresh
  rosemary
Juice of 1 lemon
½ cup granola

Per serving: Calories: 205; Total Fat: 8g; Saturated Fat: 1g; Cholesterol: 2mg; Sodium: 143mg; Potassium: 537mg; Magnesium: 47mg; Carbohydrates: 31g; Sugars: 11g; Fiber: 5g; Protein: 5g; Added Sugars: 9g; Vitamin K: 18mcg

1. Preheat the oven to 400°F. Line a baking sheet with aluminum foil or parchment paper.

2. Place the carrots, olive oil, and 1 tablespoon of honey in a rectangular dish. Add salt and pepper to taste. Toss to coat the carrots. Transfer the carrots to the prepared baking sheet and bake for 25 to 30 minutes, until slightly caramelized and golden.

3. In a bowl, combine the yogurt, rosemary, lemon juice, and remaining 1 tablespoon of honey.

4. To serve, place three or four carrots on each plate. Add a dollop of yogurt and a spoonful of granola. Serve warm.

5. If you are prepping in advance, refrigerate the yogurt mixture and carrots in separate airtight containers for 7 days. Reheat the carrots in the microwave or on the stove; then top them with yogurt and granola when ready to serve. Refrigerate the leftovers in an airtight container for up to 3 days.

PREP TIP: It's time to get crunching! For the perfect bite, make sure to cut the carrots and then dip each forkful in yogurt and coat it in granola.

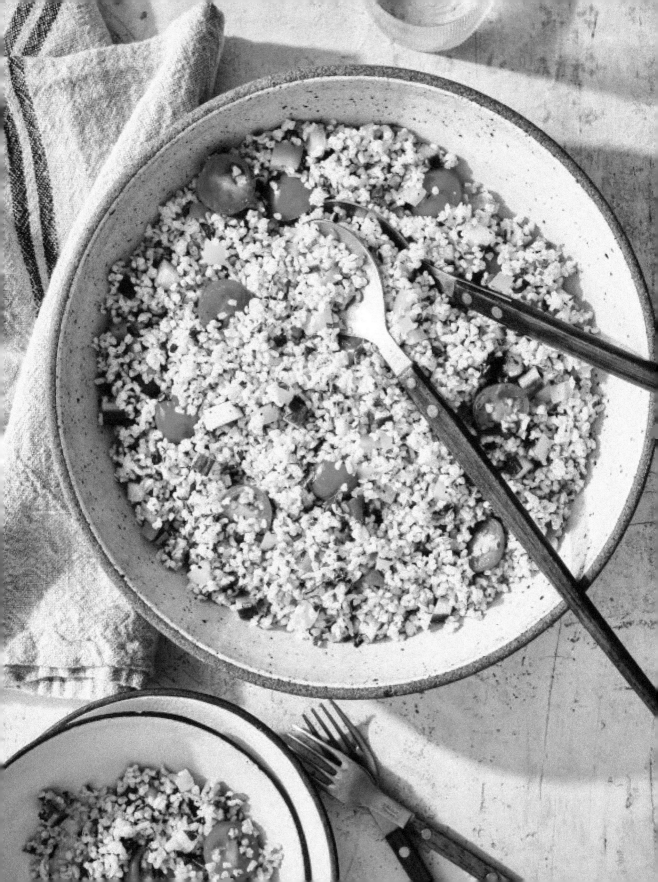

Vegetable Bulgur

Serves 6
Prep time: 5 minutes, plus 1 hour to chill / Cook time: 45 minutes
Worth the Wait

This colorful salad becomes a fiber-rich meal with the addition of bulgur, a whole grain made from cracked wheat. Just a half-cup serving of bulgur provides 3 grams of protein and is a plentiful source of B-vitamins.

2½ cups water

2 cups bulgur

2 tablespoons extra-virgin olive oil

1 small red onion, finely chopped

1 cup halved cherry tomatoes

1 yellow bell pepper, seeded and chopped

1 cucumber, chopped

½ cup loosely packed finely chopped fresh mint

½ cup loosely packed finely chopped fresh flat-leaf parsley

Grated zest and juice of 1 lemon

½ teaspoon salt

¼ teaspoon freshly ground black pepper

1. In a saucepan, bring the water to a boil over high heat; then remove it from the heat. Stir in the bulgur, cover, and let it sit until the liquid is absorbed, about 30 minutes.

2. While the bulgur cooks, heat the olive oil in a large skillet over medium heat. Add the red onion and cook for about 3 minutes, until the onion begins to soften.

3. Add the tomatoes and bell pepper and cook, stirring occasionally, for 10 to 12 minutes, until tender.

4. Stir the vegetables into the bulgur. Add the cucumber, mint, parsley, lemon zest and juice, salt, and black pepper. Stir to combine well.

5. Transfer the mixture to a container with a tight-fitting lid. Refrigerate for 1 hour before serving.

6. Refrigerate in an airtight container for up to 3 days.

PREP TIP: You can easily swap the cherry tomatoes for any tomato variety, such as Roma, or any standard medium tomato. Make sure to chop the tomatoes into even pieces for best distribution in the salad.

Per serving: Calories: 231; Total Fat: 5g; Saturated Fat: 1g; Cholesterol: 0mg; Sodium: 210mg; Potassium: 478mg; Magnesium: 98mg; Carbohydrates: 43g; Sugars: 2g; Fiber: 8g; Protein: 7g; Added Sugars: 0g; Vitamin K: 96mcg

Wild Rice with Grapes

Serves 4
Prep time: 10 minutes / Cook time: 50 minutes
5 or Fewer Ingredients
Worth the Wait

This dish has texture, a tart-sweet taste, and a hint of floral thyme. The wild rice mix can be replaced with straight wild rice or brown rice. Grapes might seem like an odd choice for a side dish, but their sweetness is lovely combined with nutty, earthy wild rice. Grapes are very high in antioxidants, including resveratrol, as well as folate, beta-carotene, manganese, iron, and vitamins A, B_1, B_2, B_6, C, E, and K. Grapes can reduce the risk of blood clots and lower both cholesterol and blood pressure. One benefit of consuming red grapes is that they contain more resveratrol in their skins than green grapes.

1 cup wild rice blend
1¾ cups water
1 teaspoon extra-virgin olive oil
2 cups red seedless grapes
2 teaspoons chopped fresh thyme
Salt
Freshly ground black pepper

Per serving: Calories: 220; Total Fat: 2g; Saturated Fat: 0g; Cholesterol: 0mg; Sodium: 43mg; Potassium: 296mg; Magnesium: 75mg; Carbohydrates: 47g; Sugars: 12g; Fiber: 3g; Protein: 5g; Added Sugars: 0g; Vitamin K: 12mcg

1. In a pot, combine the rice and water and bring to a boil over high heat. Cover, reduce the heat to low, and simmer for 45 minutes. Remove from the heat and let stand, covered, for 10 minutes. Fluff with a fork.

2. In a large skillet, heat the olive oil over medium-high heat.

3. Add the grapes and thyme and sauté until the grapes begin to burst, about 5 minutes.

4. Stir in the wild rice mixture and season with salt and pepper. Serve.

5. Refrigerate the leftovers in an airtight container for 4 to 5 days.

PREP TIP: Wild rice is not rice at all; it is the seed of a water grass that is indigenous to North America. You can find both cultivated and authentic handpicked wild rice in your local store. Cultivated wild rice is less expensive and has a milder taste and dark ebony color. It will work fine in this recipe and is usually the type found in premixed rice blends.

Easy Italian-Inspired Roasted Vegetables

DAIRY-FREE
VEGETARIAN

Serves 6
Prep time: 15 minutes / Cook time: 45 minutes
Worth the Wait

Crusty bread is perfect for dipping into this colorful vegetable mélange, inspired by Italian staples including Roma tomatoes, eggplant, and zucchini. The natural sauce this dish makes is incredible. And you'll get plenty of fiber in this tasty dish (7 grams per serving). Once you make this dish twice, you'll be throwing it together during your next family dinner.

Nonstick cooking spray
2 eggplants, peeled and cut into ⅛-inch-thick slices
1 zucchini, cut into ¼-inch-thick slices
1 yellow summer squash, cut into ¼-inch-thick slices
2 Roma tomatoes, cut into ⅛-inch-thick slices
¼ cup extra-virgin olive oil, plus 2 tablespoons
1 tablespoon garlic powder
¼ teaspoon dried oregano
¼ teaspoon dried basil
¼ teaspoon salt
Freshly ground black pepper

1. Preheat the oven to 400°F.

2. In a large bowl, toss the eggplant, zucchini, squash, and tomatoes with 2 tablespoons of the olive oil, the garlic powder, oregano, basil, salt, and pepper to taste.

3. Spray a 9 x 13-inch baking dish with cooking spray. In the dish, alternate layers of eggplant, zucchini, squash, and tomato. Drizzle the top with the remaining ¼ cup of olive oil.

4. Bake, uncovered, for 40 to 45 minutes, or until the vegetables are golden brown.

5. Refrigerate the leftovers in an airtight container for 3 to 5 days.

PREP TIP: For a sweet note, consider adding sautéed shallots or roasted red bell peppers.

Per serving: Calories: 186; Total Fat: 14g; Saturated Fat: 2g; Cholesterol: 0mg; Sodium: 108mg; Potassium: 659mg; Magnesium: 41mg; Carbohydrates: 15g; Sugars: 9g; Fiber: 7g; Protein: 3g; Added Sugars: 0g; Vitamin K: 20mcg

Braised Sweet Peppers

Serves 4
Prep time: 10 minutes / Cook time: 40 minutes
Worth the Wait

Bell peppers are very low in calories and are an excellent source of vitamins and antioxidants. To best preserve the healthy benefits of peppers, I suggest braising them. When braising, the vegetables are cooked "low and slow" in a flavorful liquid such as broth or wine. You will also find that braising vegetables intensifies their flavor. After trying these peppers, braise carrots, fennel, and even cabbage. You are in for a delicious treat!

¼ cup extra-virgin olive oil

1 red onion, thinly sliced

3 red bell peppers, seeded and cut into 1-inch strips

3 green bell peppers, seeded and cut into 1-inch strips

2 garlic cloves, chopped

¼ teaspoon cayenne pepper

⅛ teaspoon salt

⅛ teaspoon freshly ground black pepper

¼ cup vegetable broth

1 tablespoon chopped fresh thyme

1. In a large saucepan, heat the olive oil over medium heat.

2. Add the red onion and cook for 5 minutes.

3. Add the red and green bell peppers, garlic, cayenne, salt, and black pepper.

4. Pour in the vegetable broth and bring the mixture to a boil. Cover the pan and reduce the heat to low. Cook for 35 minutes, stirring occasionally, until the vegetables are soft but still firm.

5. Sprinkle the peppers with the thyme and serve.

6. Refrigerate the leftovers in an airtight container for 3 to 5 days.

SUBSTITUTION TIP: Use 1 teaspoon of dried thyme instead of fresh and add it when you add the cayenne.

Per serving: Calories: 179; Total Fat: 14g; Saturated Fat: 2g; Cholesterol: 0mg; Sodium: 85mg; Potassium: 397mg; Magnesium: 24mg; Carbohydrates: 13g; Sugars: 7g; Fiber: 4g; Protein: 2g; Added Sugars: 0g; Vitamin K: 19mcg

Caramelized Sweet Potato Wedges

DAIRY-FREE
VEGETARIAN

Serves 4
Prep time: 15 minutes / Cook time: 40 minutes
5 or Fewer Ingredients
Worth the Wait

Sweet potato fries are a beloved staple in restaurants, where they're typically deep-fried. This version features fresh sweet potatoes sliced into wedges, coated in olive oil, and roasted at a high temperature until crispy on the outside and tender on the inside. Serve them as a snack or as a side dish to make a complete meal.

Nonstick cooking spray
2 sweet potatoes, cut
    into ½-inch wedges
2 tablespoons
    extra-virgin olive oil
¼ teaspoon salt
¼ teaspoon ground
    black pepper

Per serving: Calories: 116; Total Fat: 7g; Saturated Fat: 1g; Cholesterol: 0mg; Sodium: 181mg; Potassium: 219mg; Magnesium: 16mg; Carbohydrates: 13g; Sugars: 3g; Fiber: 2g; Protein: 1g; Added Sugars: 0g; Vitamin K: 5mcg

1. Preheat the oven to 450°F. Line a baking sheet with a wire rack and coat it with cooking spray.

2. Evenly coat the sweet potatoes in olive oil and season with the salt and pepper.

3. Line up the wedges on the wire rack, about 1 inch apart, and roast for 30 to 35 minutes. Turn the oven to a low broil or 400°F for 3 to 4 minutes, until the edges of the sweet potato wedges are slightly browned. Serve once they have slightly cooled.

4. Refrigerate the leftovers in an airtight container for 3 to 5 days. To reheat the potato wedges, line them up on a baking sheet with a wire rack and roast at 450°F for 5 to 6 minutes, until crispy again.

PREP TIP: You can add unique flavors to these wedges by tossing them with a tablespoon of garam masala, Italian seasoning, or chili powder.

SUBSTITUTION TIP: Try Yukon Gold or red potatoes instead of sweet potatoes.

Stuffed Cherry Tomatoes

VEGETARIAN
QUICK

Serves 8
Prep time: 15 minutes
5 or Fewer Ingredients

These pretty little pop-in-your-mouth treats make great party appetizers. Kids love their fresh summery flavor, too. The lycopene in tomatoes is a powerful antioxidant that helps protect the skin from harmful UV rays. In addition, lycopene is notable for its heart-protective qualities.

24 cherry tomatoes
⅓ cup part-skim ricotta cheese
¼ cup chopped peeled cucumber
1 tablespoon finely chopped red onion
2 teaspoons minced fresh basil

1. Slice off the top of each tomato. Carefully scrape out and discard the pulp inside.

2. In a bowl, combine the ricotta, cucumber, red onion, and basil. Stir well.

3. Spoon the ricotta cheese mixture into the tomatoes and serve cold.

4. Store leftovers in an airtight container for 3 to 4 days.

PREP TIP: The tomatoes can be stuffed, covered, and refrigerated for up to 1 hour before serving.

Per serving (3 tomatoes): Calories: 25; Total Fat: 1g; Saturated Fat: 1g; Cholesterol: 3mg; Sodium: 13mg; Potassium: 145mg; Magnesium: 9mg; Carbohydrates: 3g; Sugars: 1g; Fiber: 1g; Protein: 2g; Added Sugars: 0g; Vitamin K: 7mcg

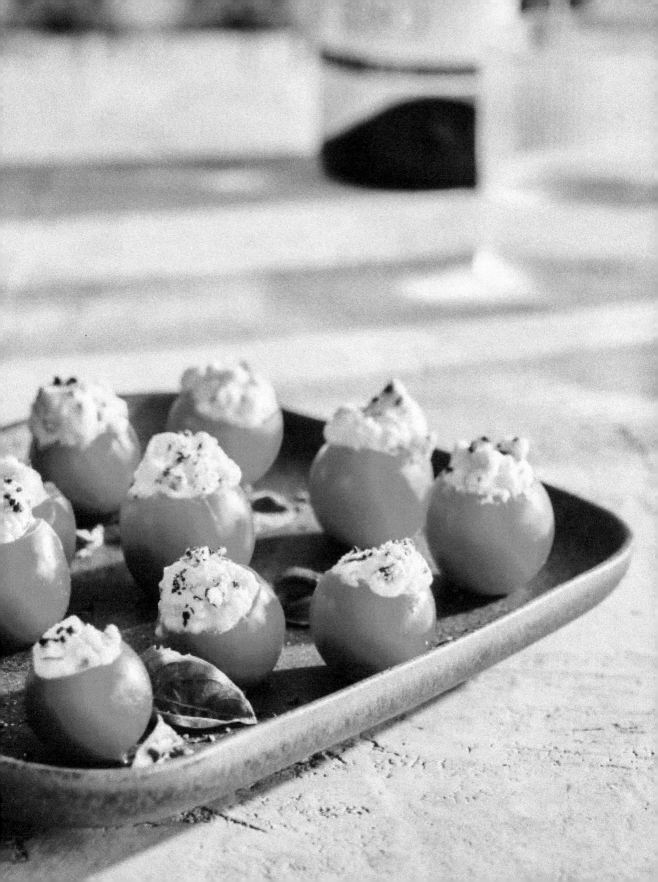

Turmeric-Spiced Crispy Cauliflower

Serves 4
Prep time: 5 minutes / Cook time: 30 minutes
5 or Fewer Ingredients

Cauliflower is one of the most versatile vegetables out there. In this recipe it's roasted with a variety of spices, including turmeric, which adds a beautiful golden glow and provides powerful anti-inflammatory properties. Black pepper enhances its antioxidant effects.

1 head cauliflower, cut into florets
1 tablespoon extra-virgin olive oil
2 teaspoons ground turmeric
1 teaspoon ground cumin
½ teaspoon ground cayenne pepper
Kosher salt
Freshly ground black pepper

1. Preheat the oven to 400°F. Line a rimmed baking sheet with aluminum foil or parchment paper.

2. In a large mixing bowl, combine the cauliflower, olive oil, turmeric, cumin, and cayenne pepper. Add salt and black pepper to taste. Toss until evenly coated, and transfer to the prepared baking sheet.

3. Bake for 25 to 30 minutes, until the cauliflower is browned and slightly crispy.

4. Refrigerate in an airtight container for up to 4 days.

PREP TIP: You can make cauliflower soup by following this recipe and then pureeing the roasted florets in the blender with 4 cups of vegetable stock. Serve the soup hot or cold.

Per serving: Calories: 74; Total Fat: 4g; Saturated Fat: 1g; Cholesterol: 0mg; Sodium: 84mg; Potassium: 485mg; Magnesium: 27mg; Carbohydrates: 9g; Sugars: 3g; Fiber: 3g; Protein: 3g; Added Sugars: 0g; Vitamin K: 25mcg

Tabbouleh

Serves 4 to 6
Prep time: 15 minutes / Cook time: 15 minutes

This is a quick and easy version of a classic Mediterranean staple, sure to brighten any plate. Tabbouleh is a national dish of Lebanon, but variations can be found in almost every country on the Mediterranean Sea. You can put together this salad in a snap with ingredients you probably already have in the kitchen. Cooking the bulgur takes the most time, so do this ahead and store it in an airtight container in the refrigerator for up to 4 days.

1 cup water
½ cup dried bulgur
½ English cucumber, quartered lengthwise and sliced
2 tomatoes on the vine, diced
2 scallions, green part only, chopped
Juice of 1 lemon
2 cups coarsely chopped fresh Italian parsley
⅓ cup coarsely chopped fresh mint leaves
1 garlic clove
¼ cup extra-virgin olive oil
Salt
Freshly ground black pepper

1. In a medium saucepan, combine the water and bulgur and bring to a boil over high heat. Reduce the heat to low, cover, and cook until the bulgur is tender, about 12 minutes. Drain the bulgur, fluff it with a fork, and set it aside to cool.

2. In a large bowl, toss together the bulgur, cucumber, tomatoes, scallions, and lemon juice.

3. In a food processor, combine the parsley, mint, and garlic and process until finely chopped.

4. Add the chopped herb mixture to the bulgur mixture and stir to combine. Add the olive oil and stir to incorporate.

5. Season with salt and pepper and serve.

6. Refrigerate leftover tabbouleh in an airtight container for up to 4 days.

PREP TIP: Tabbouleh is great stuffed inside cooked vegetables, like tomatoes, for a vegetarian main meal.

Per serving: Calories: 223; Total Fat: 14g; Saturated Fat: 2g; Cholesterol: 0mg; Sodium: 70mg; Potassium: 545mg; Magnesium: 67mg; Carbohydrates: 23g; Sugars: 4g; Fiber: 5g; Protein: 5g; Added Sugars: 0g; Vitamin K: 567mcg

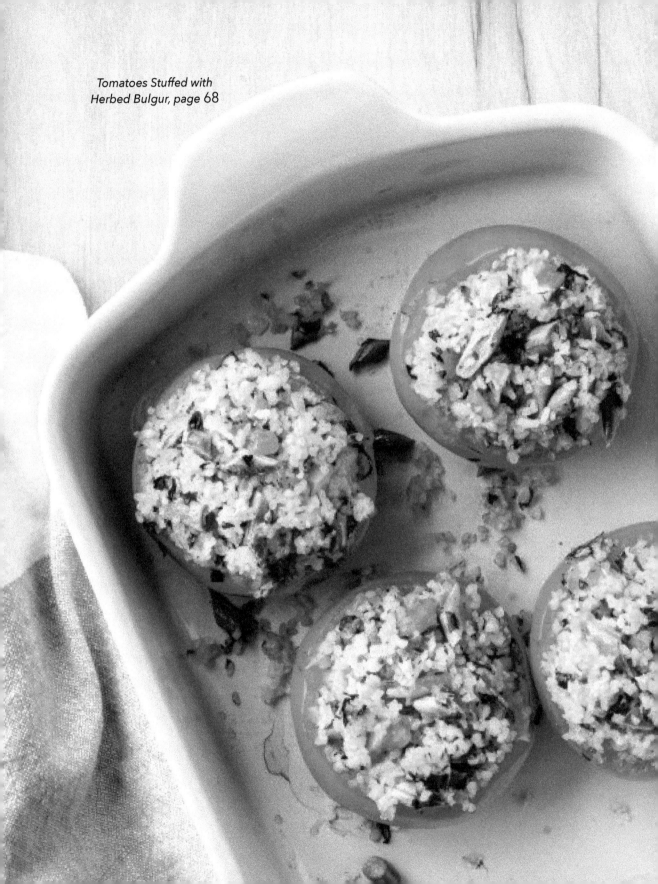

*Tomatoes Stuffed with
Herbed Bulgur, page 68*

Chapter 5

Vegetarian Mains

Tomatoes Stuffed with Herbed Bulgur

Serves 4
Prep time: 10 minutes / Cook time: 40 minutes
Worth the Wait

Stuffed vegetables can be found in many Mediterranean countries, such as France, Spain, Greece, and Italy. The preparation is easy and versatile, and almost any ingredients can be combined and spooned into tomatoes, so use your imagination. This combination is effective because green beans and tomatoes create optimal iron absorption to boost muscle and brain health. Iron is crucial for the production of hemoglobin, which is the mode of transport for oxygen throughout the body.

1 cup bulgur

2 cups water

4 large tomatoes

1 tablespoon extra-virgin olive oil

½ sweet onion, finely chopped

2 teaspoons minced garlic

2 cups green beans, cut into ½-inch pieces

2 tablespoons chopped fresh parsley

1 tablespoon chopped fresh basil

1 tablespoon chopped fresh oregano

Grated zest and juice of 1 lemon

Salt

Freshly ground black pepper

1. In a small pot, combine the bulgur and water. Bring to a boil over high heat, cover, and reduce the heat to low to simmer until tender, about 15 minutes. Drain the bulgur and set it aside.

2. Preheat the oven to 400°F.

3. Cut the tops off the tomatoes and scoop out the pulp and seeds with a spoon. Place the tomato shells, cut-side up, into a 9 x 9-inch baking dish and set aside. Chop the pulp and seeds coarsely, and transfer them to a bowl.

4. In a medium skillet, heat the olive oil over medium heat. Sauté the onion and garlic until softened, about 3 minutes. Stir in the tomato pulp, green beans, parsley, basil, oregano, and lemon zest and juice. Sauté for 1 minute and remove from the heat.

5. Stir in the cooked bulgur and toss to combine. Season with salt and pepper. Spoon the bulgur mixture into the tomatoes and bake until the tomatoes are very soft, about 20 minutes. Serve.

6. Refrigerate in an airtight container for 3 to 4 days.

SUBSTITUTION TIP: Stuffed vegetables are incredibly versatile, so they can be prepared to suit any diet or allergy issue. If gluten is a concern, try black beans, lentils, quinoa, or even riced cauliflower in place of the bulgur.

Per serving: Calories: 209; Total Fat: 4g; Saturated Fat: 1g; Cholesterol: 0mg; Sodium: 59mg; Potassium: 731mg; Magnesium: 94mg; Carbohydrates: 40g; Sugars: 7g; Fiber: 8g; Protein: 7g; Added Sugars: 0g; Vitamin K: 58mcg

Freekeh Salad with Arugula and Peaches

Serves 4
Prep time: 10 minutes / Cook time: 20 minutes

Keep your salads exciting by varying your leafy green and whole grains. Make them colorful by adding fresh fruit to provide a touch of sweetness. This salad is made unique and exciting with freekeh, peaches, and arugula.

1¼ cups water
⅛ teaspoon salt, plus
  ¼ teaspoon
½ cup freekeh
2 tablespoons
  champagne vinegar
3 tablespoons
  extra-virgin olive oil
2 teaspoons honey
1 tablespoon lemon
  juice
Freshly ground black
  pepper
5 ounces arugula
2 ripe peaches, pitted
  and sliced
¼ cup slivered almonds
⅓ cup Pecorino
  Romano, cut into
  slivers

1. In a medium saucepan over medium heat, bring the water and ⅛ teaspoon of salt to a boil. Add the freekeh, cover, and reduce the heat to medium-low. Simmer for 15 minutes, or until the liquid is absorbed.

2. In a small mixing bowl, whisk together the vinegar, olive oil, honey, lemon juice, and remaining ¼ teaspoon of salt. Add pepper to taste.

3. Place the arugula, peaches, and cooked freekeh in a large serving bowl. Drizzle with the dressing and toss gently. Add the almonds and Pecorino Romano just before serving.

4. If you know you will be saving some salad for later, refrigerate it with the dressing stored separately in an airtight container for up to 5 days. It's best to consume salad that's been dressed the same day as the acids in the dressing will easily wilt the leafy greens.

SUBSTITUTION TIP: You can use any whole grain in this salad—barley and wheat berries are two great substitutes for freekeh. Use quinoa for a gluten-free option.

Per serving: Calories: 273; Total Fat: 16g; Saturated Fat: 3g; Cholesterol: 9mg; Sodium: 213mg; Potassium: 413mg; Magnesium: 74mg; Carbohydrates: 27g; Sugars: 7g; Fiber: 5g; Protein: 8g; Added Sugars: 3g; Vitamin K: 47mcg

Greek Bean Soup

DAIRY-FREE
VEGETARIAN
1 POT MEAL

Serves: 4
Prep time: 10 minutes / Cook time: 35 minutes
Worth the Wait

Some say this is the national dish of Greece, and in some parts of the country, there are competitions to determine the best recipe. This simple, healthy, and delicious bean soup will warm you on a cold day and keep you full. The soup is vegan, but if you don't follow a vegan diet, try adding a sprinkle of feta when you serve it.

2 tablespoons extra-virgin olive oil
1 large onion, chopped
1 (15-ounce) can diced tomatoes
1 (15-ounce) can Great Northern beans, drained and rinsed
2 celery stalks, chopped
2 carrots, cut into long ribbons
⅓ teaspoon chopped fresh thyme
¼ cup chopped fresh Italian parsley
1 bay leaf
Salt
Freshly ground black pepper

1. In a Dutch oven, heat the olive oil over medium-high heat. Add the onion and sauté for 4 minutes, or until softened. Add the tomatoes with the juices, beans, celery, carrots, thyme, parsley, and bay leaf, and then add water to cover the mixture by about 2 inches.

2. Bring the soup to a boil, reduce the heat to low, cover, and simmer for 30 minutes, or until the vegetables are tender.

3. Remove the bay leaf, season with salt and pepper, and serve.

4. Refrigerate the leftovers in an airtight container for up to 4 days.

PREP TIP: You may need to add more water during the cooking process; for more flavor, use vegetable broth instead.

Per serving: Calories: 187; Total Fat: 7g; Saturated Fat: 1g; Cholesterol: 0mg; Sodium: 203mg; Potassium: 688mg; Magnesium: 55mg; Carbohydrates: 25g; Sugars: 6g; Fiber: 9g; Protein: 7g; Added Sugars: 0g; Vitamin K: 78mcg

Vegetable Tagine

Serves 4
Prep time: 15 minutes / Cook time: 45 minutes
Worth the Wait

In North African cooking, tagines tend to be a mix of vegetables (or meat), fruit, and spices, but the word "tagine" refers to both the dish and the vessel in which it is cooked. A traditional tagine is a clay or ceramic pot with a cone-shaped lid that traps and condenses liquid that evaporates from the ingredients so you don't lose a single delicious drop. Using a stockpot with a lid mimics this process. This recipe is a winning combination that surprises many diners and keeps them coming back for more.

3 tablespoons
   extra-virgin olive oil
1 onion, thinly sliced
5 garlic cloves, minced
2 carrots, cut into long
   ribbons
2 red bell peppers,
   seeded and coarsely
   chopped
1 (15-ounce) can diced
   tomatoes
½ cup chopped dried
   apricots
1 to 2 tablespoons
   harissa
1 teaspoon ground
   coriander
½ teaspoon ground
   turmeric
½ teaspoon ground
   cinnamon

Ingredients continued on page 73

1. In a large stockpot, heat the olive oil over medium-high heat. Add the onion and garlic and sauté for 5 minutes. Add the carrots and bell peppers and sauté for 7 to 10 minutes, until the vegetables are tender.

2. Add the tomatoes, apricots, harissa, coriander, turmeric, and cinnamon and cook for 5 minutes. Add the broth and sweet potato and bring to a boil. Reduce the heat to low, cover, and simmer for 20 minutes, or until the sweet potato is tender.

3 cups vegetable broth

1 sweet potato, peeled and cubed

1 (15-ounce) can chickpeas, drained and rinsed

Salt

Freshly ground black pepper

3. Add the chickpeas and simmer for 3 minutes to heat through. Season with salt and pepper and serve.

4. Refrigerate the leftovers in an airtight container for up to 4 days.

PREP TIP: Feel free to change up the vegetables. This tagine is a delicious way to clear out any produce left in your refrigerator.

Per serving: Calories: 324; Total Fat: 12g; Saturated Fat: 2g; Cholesterol: 0mg; Sodium: 210mg; Potassium: 968mg; Magnesium: 69mg; Carbohydrates: 48g; Sugars: 21g; Fiber: 12g; Protein: 9g; Added Sugars: 0g; Vitamin K: 20mcg

Lentil Burgers

Serves 4 to 6
Prep time: 15 minutes / Cook time: 15 minutes

Enjoy a savory burger without the cholesterol and saturated fat you'll get in a meat burger. This burger is packed with fiber-rich lentils and cremini mushrooms, a plant food rich in vitamin D. Seasoned with garlic, miso, and smoked paprika, it may just be the best veggie burger you've ever made!

1 cup cooked green lentils, divided
½ cup low-fat plain Greek yogurt
Grated zest and juice of ½ lemon
½ teaspoon garlic powder, divided
⅛ teaspoon salt
6 ounces cremini mushrooms, finely chopped
3 tablespoons extra-virgin olive oil, divided
¼ teaspoon white miso
¼ teaspoon smoked paprika
¼ cup gluten-free flour
3 pitas, halved

1. In a blender, pour in ½ cup of lentils and partially puree them until somewhat smooth but with many whole lentils still remaining.

2. In a small bowl, combine the yogurt, lemon zest and juice, ¼ teaspoon of garlic powder, and the salt. Set aside.

3. In a medium bowl, combine the mushrooms, 2 tablespoons of the olive oil, miso, paprika, and the remaining ¼ teaspoon of garlic powder. Add the lentils and stir. Vigorously stir in flour until the mixture holds together when squeezed; if it doesn't, continue to mash the lentils until it does and add 1 or 2 tablespoons more of flour if needed. Form into 6 roughly ¾-inch-thick patties.

4. In a large nonstick sauté pan or skillet, heat the remaining 1 tablespoon of olive oil over medium heat. Working in batches, place the patties in the skillet and cook until they are deeply browned and very crisp on the bottom side, about 3 minutes. Carefully turn and repeat on the second side, adding more oil as needed to maintain a light coating around the patties in skillet. Repeat with the remaining patties, adding more oil to the pan if needed.

5. Spread the yogurt mixture into the pita halves when ready to serve. Then add one patty into each pocket.

6. Make ahead of time and refrigerate the uncooked patties for a day, or freeze them by stacking them between parchment paper in a freezer-friendly zip-top bag or airtight container for up to 3 months. Thaw in the refrigerator and heat the patties according to the instructions in step 4. Refrigerate any leftover cooked lentil burgers in an airtight container for 3 to 4 days.

SUBSTITUTION TIP: To make this lentil burger dairy-free, swap out the Greek yogurt for an equal amount of hummus. Look for mild versions of hummus made simply with chickpeas, tahini, lemon, and salt.

Per serving: Calories: 343; Total Fat: 12g; Saturated Fat: 2g; Cholesterol: 2mg; Sodium: 329mg; Potassium: 549mg; Magnesium: 65mg; Carbohydrates: 49g; Sugars: 4g; Fiber: 8g; Protein: 12g; Added Sugars: 0g; Vitamin K: 8mcg

Black-Eyed Peas and Kale Bowl

Serves 4
Prep time: 10 minutes / Cook time: 20 minutes

Boost your bone health with this dish of black-eyed peas and kale. Black-eyed peas are a source of plant-based calcium (106 milligrams per ½-cup serving). Kale has a decent amount of calcium, too. Serve this dish with a couple pieces of oven-warmed naan to scoop up every last bite.

½ cup brown rice
1 tablespoon extra-virgin olive oil
½ sweet onion, finely chopped
2 teaspoons minced garlic
2 (15-ounce) cans black-eyed peas, drained and rinsed
2 cups stemmed and sliced fresh kale
2 large tomatoes, finely chopped
3 tablespoons finely chopped chives

Per serving: Calories: 322; Total Fat: 5g; Saturated Fat: 1g; Cholesterol: 0mg; Sodium: 14mg; Potassium: 838mg; Magnesium: 143mg; Carbohydrates: 57g; Sugars: 5g; Fiber: 14g; Protein: 15g; Added Sugars: 0g; Vitamin K: 71mcg

1. Cook the rice according to the package instructions and set aside. You can do this up to 3 days ahead, storing the rice in a sealed container in the refrigerator.

2. In a large skillet, heat the olive oil over medium-high heat.

3. Sauté the onion and garlic until softened, about 3 minutes.

4. Stir in the black-eyed peas and rice and cook until heated through, about 10 minutes.

5. Stir in the kale and sauté until wilted, about 5 minutes.

6. Spoon the mixture into four bowls and then divide the tomatoes among the bowls.

7. Serve topped with chives.

8. Refrigerate the leftovers in an airtight container for 4 to 5 days.

PREP TIP: Bowls are a trendy presentation found in lots of eateries, from small diners to Michelin-rated restaurants. A bowl is an assortment of ingredients, usually along a similar theme, combined in one dish and eaten together. Sliced avocado, red bell pepper, and chunks of canned or fresh-cooked salmon would be great additions to this fresh and satisfying meal.

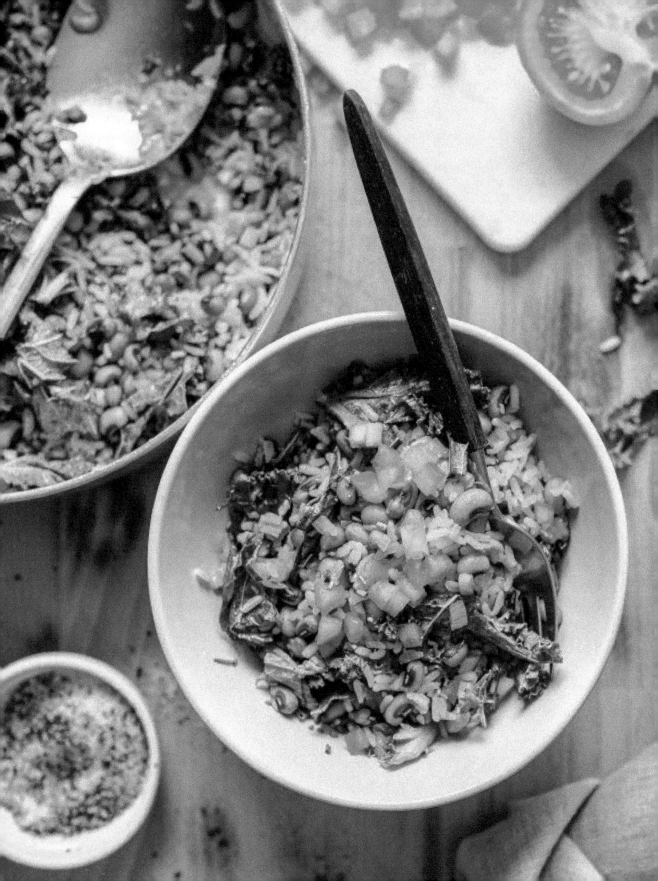

Falafel in Pita

Serves 4
Prep time: 25 minutes / Cook time: 40 minutes
Worth the Wait

Falafel are chickpea patties that originated in Egypt and remain popular all over the Middle East. They are usually deep-fried, but they can also be baked. Dress them up with tzatziki and stuff them in a pita for a classic Mediterranean sandwich.

**3 tablespoons
extra-virgin olive oil,
divided, plus more for
brushing**
1 cup dried chickpeas
**1 medium onion,
roughly chopped**
2 garlic cloves, peeled
**3 tablespoons chopped
fresh flat-leaf parsley**
**1 tablespoon
all-purpose flour**
**1 teaspoon ground
coriander**
**1 teaspoon
ground cumin**
½ teaspoon salt
**⅛ teaspoon cayenne
pepper**
4 pita breads
**½ head iceberg
lettuce, chopped**

1. Preheat the oven to 350°F. Line a rimmed baking sheet with parchment paper and lightly brush the parchment with olive oil.

2. Put the chickpeas in a pot and cover them with water. Bring to a boil over high heat; then reduce the heat to low and simmer for 15 minutes. Drain the chickpeas and let cool.

3. In a food processor, combine the onion, garlic, parsley, flour, 1 tablespoon of olive oil, the coriander, cumin, salt, and cayenne. Pulse a few times to combine. Add the chickpeas and process to form a thick paste.

4. Scoop out about 1 tablespoon of the falafel mixture, roll it in your hands to create a ball, and then flatten it into a patty about 2 inches wide. You should get 12 to 15 patties. Place the patties on the prepared baking sheet.

5. Brush the patties with the remaining 2 tablespoons of olive oil. Bake for 15 minutes. Flip and bake for 10 minutes more, or until lightly browned.

Ingredients continued on page 79

1 tomato, chopped

1 red onion, chopped

¼ cup Greek
Cucumber-Yogurt Dip/
Tzatziki (page 134)

6. Place three falafel in each pita pocket. Top with lettuce, tomato, red onion, and a dollop of tzatziki.

7. Refrigerate the leftover falafel in an airtight container for 2 to 4 days. If you are prepping in advance, you can refrigerate uncooked falafel patties for up to 4 days.

SUBSTITUTION TIP: Cilantro makes a great swap for the parsley since it has a similar look and texture and has notes of citrus, floral, and slight peppery appeal. It can brighten the overall flavor a bit more.

Per serving: Calories: 506; Total Fat: 15g; Saturated Fat: 2g; Cholesterol: 2mg; Sodium: 648mg; Potassium: 776mg; Magnesium: 77mg; Carbohydrates: 77g; Sugars: 12g; Fiber: 10g; Protein: 18g; Added Sugars: 0g; Vitamin K: 83mcg

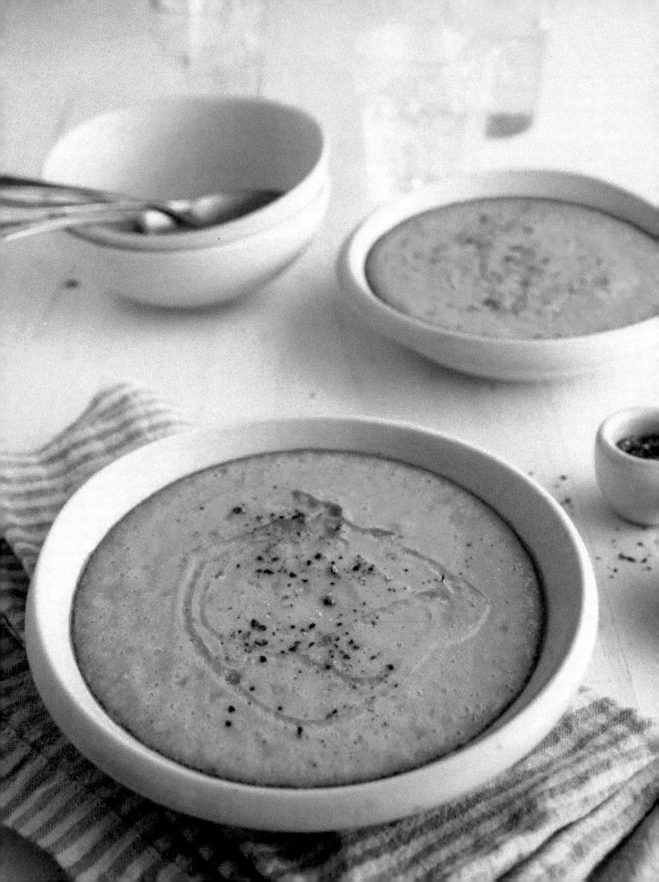

Fresh Gazpacho Soup

Serves 6 to 8
Prep time: 15 minutes, plus 2 hours to chill

Gazpacho is full of fresh flavors and is a great way to get in more veggies. Because it involves no cooking, this is one of the easiest soups to make. This soup originated in Spain, and there are many variations of it. Low in calories and high in flavor, gazpacho makes an ideal healthy snack or side dish.

½ cup water

2 slices white bread, crust removed

2 pounds ripe tomatoes, cored and chopped

1 Persian cucumber, peeled and chopped

1 clove garlic, finely chopped

⅓ cup extra-virgin olive oil, plus more for garnish

2 tablespoons red wine vinegar

1 teaspoon salt

½ teaspoon freshly ground black pepper

1. Soak the bread in the water for 5 minutes; discard water when done.

2. Blend the bread, tomatoes, cucumber, garlic, olive oil, vinegar, salt, and pepper in a food processor or blender until completely smooth.

3. Pour the soup into a glass container and store it in the refrigerator until completely chilled, approximately 2 hours and up to overnight.

4. When you are ready to serve, pour the soup into a bowl and top it with a drizzle of olive oil.

5. Refrigerate the soup in an airtight container for 4 to 5 days.

PREP TIP: You can also serve the soup topped with fresh herbs, such as basil, parsley, or thyme. I also like to add half an onion or a green or red bell pepper for a little sweetness. Add these variations when blending the other ingredients.

Per serving: Calories: 164; Total Fat: 12g; Saturated Fat: 2g; Cholesterol: 0mg; Sodium: 441mg; Potassium: 448mg; Magnesium: 26mg; Carbohydrates: 12g; Sugars: 5g; Fiber: 2g; Protein: 3g; Added Sugars: 0g; Vitamin K: 28mcg

Roasted Root Vegetable Grain Bowls

VEGETARIAN

Serves 4
Prep time: 10 minutes / Cook time: 30 minutes

Root vegetables are perfect for vegetarian meals. Roasting brings out their sweetness, and they pair nicely with hearty grains such as sorghum, making this bowl a fiber-rich meal.

1 (8-ounce) package white or baby bella mushrooms, quartered

2 turnips, peeled and cut into half-moons

2 large carrots, peeled and sliced

1 golden beet, cut into ½-inch cubes

1 red beet, cut into ½-inch cubes

1 cup uncooked pearled sorghum

Salt

Freshly ground black pepper

1 tablespoon extra-virgin olive oil

4 teaspoons balsamic vinegar

½ cup crumbled goat cheese

Fresh rosemary, stripped from stems, for garnish (optional)

1. Preheat the oven to 400°F.

2. On a large baking sheet, arrange the mushrooms, turnips, carrots, and golden and red beets in a single layer. Roast for 25 to 30 minutes, or until fully cooked. Remove the mushrooms early if needed to prevent burning.

3. Meanwhile, in a medium saucepan, cook the sorghum in water according to the package instructions, simmering for 15 to 20 minutes, or until all the liquid is absorbed. Remove from the heat, fluff with a fork, and season with salt and pepper.

4. To serve, distribute the roasted vegetables and mushrooms evenly among four plates. Add the cooked sorghum on top, and drizzle with the olive oil and balsamic vinegar. Top with the goat cheese and rosemary (if using), and serve.

5. Refrigerate leftover grain bowls in an airtight container for up to 5 days.

PREP TIP: Look for sorghum in the health section or bulk bins in your grocery store. You could also order online or substitute with grains like farro, freekeh, or Israeli couscous.

Per serving: Calories: 292; Total Fat: 8g; Saturated Fat: 3g; Cholesterol: 7mg; Sodium: 207mg; Potassium: 729mg; Magnesium: 108mg; Carbohydrates: 49g; Sugars: 10g; Fiber: 7g; Protein: 11g; Added Sugars: 0g; Vitamin K: 7mcg

White Bean and Kale Skillet with Quick-Fried Egg

Serves 4
Prep time: 5 minutes / Cook time: 25 minutes

Whether you start or end your day with this meal, you'll be getting a healthy dose of both protein and fiber to keep you satisfied.

2 tablespoons
extra-virgin olive oil,
divided
1 tablespoon
low-sodium soy sauce
1 (8-ounce) package
tempeh, cut into
cubes
1 large bunch kale,
shredded
1 garlic clove, minced
Pinch salt
Freshly ground black
pepper
¼ teaspoon red
pepper flakes
1 (15.5-ounce) can
cannellini beans,
drained and rinsed
4 large eggs

Per serving: Calories: 355;
Total Fat: 19g; Saturated
Fat: 4g; Cholesterol: 186mg;
Sodium: 270mg; Potassium:
907mg; Magnesium: 119mg;
Carbohydrates: 26g; Sugars:
2g; Fiber: 7g; Protein:
26g; Added Sugars: 0g;
Vitamin K: 476mcg

1. In a large skillet, heat 1 tablespoon of olive oil and the soy sauce over medium-high heat. Add the tempeh, and stir until coated. Allow to cook until the tempeh begins to crisp, 5 to 8 minutes, stirring occasionally.

2. Transfer the tempeh to a plate and cover it to keep the tempeh warm.

3. In the same skillet, heat the remaining 1 tablespoon of olive oil over medium-high heat. Add the kale, garlic, salt and pepper to taste, and red pepper flakes. Cook, covered, for 5 to 6 minutes, or until the kale softens and becomes a dark, vibrant green color. Stir in the beans and heat through, cooking uncovered for about 3 minutes more.

4. Divide the kale mixture evenly among four bowls, and top with the cooked tempeh. In the same skillet over medium-high heat, prepare the quick-fried eggs (cooked over-easy to over-medium). Top each bowl with one egg and serve immediately.

5. Make ahead and refrigerate for up to 5 days. It's best to prepare the egg just before serving.

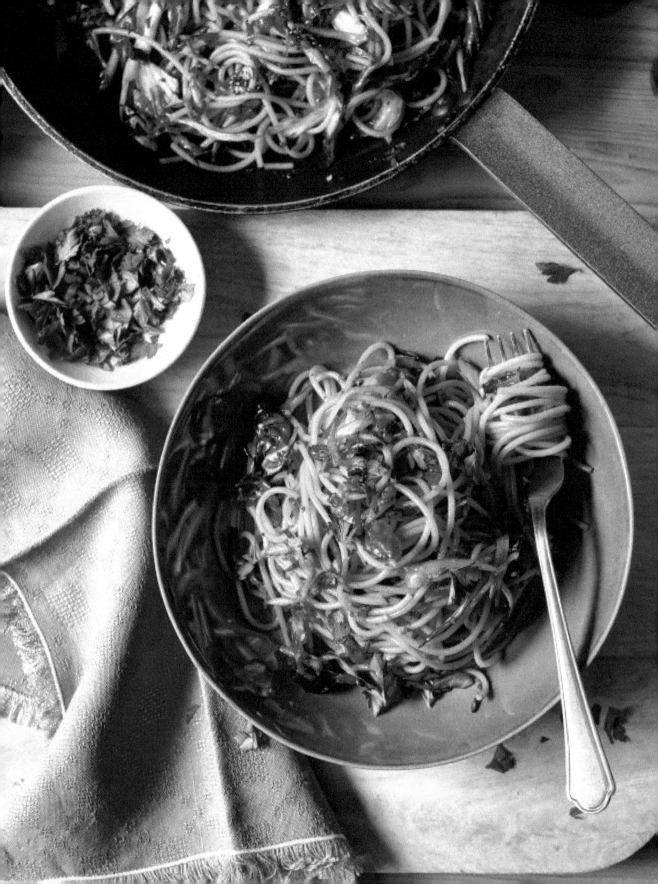

Spaghetti with Braised Balsamic Vinegar Radicchio

DAIRY-FREE
VEGETARIAN

Serves 4
Prep time: 10 minutes / Cook time: 20 minutes

You don't have to stick with broccoli, peas, or mushrooms to add veggies to your pasta. Braised radicchio keeps this dish veggie-ful and unique. The hot chili flakes, bitter radicchio, tart balsamic, and nutty pasta combine to create a solid and satisfying meal. The deep red color of the radicchio accented by the fresh green parsley is visually fabulous.

8 ounces dry spaghetti
2 tablespoons extra-virgin olive oil
1 tablespoon minced garlic
2 heads radicchio, shredded
¼ cup balsamic vinegar
Pinch red pepper flakes
Salt, for seasoning
2 tablespoons finely chopped fresh parsley

Per serving: Calories: 295; Total Fat: 8g; Saturated Fat: 1g; Cholesterol: 0mg; Sodium: 54mg; Potassium: 254mg; Magnesium: 37mg; Carbohydrates: 47g; Sugars: 4g; Fiber: 2g; Protein: 8g; Added Sugars: 0g; Vitamin K: 112mcg

1. Cook the pasta according to the package instructions.

2. While the pasta is cooking, heat the olive oil in a large skillet over medium-high heat.

3. Sauté the garlic until softened, about 2 minutes.

4. Add the shredded radicchio and sauté until tender, 6 to 7 minutes.

5. Stir in the balsamic vinegar and red pepper flakes and sauté 3 to 4 minutes more.

6. Add the cooked pasta and toss to coat.

7. Season with salt and serve topped with parsley.

8. Refrigerate the leftovers in an airtight container for up to 7 days.

PREP TIP: The color of radicchio is glorious. It's also quite delicate, so this vegetable should only be stored for about 3 days after being purchased. For the best results, find compact heads of radicchio with no withered, limp, or yellowed leaves. Cut out the core if the head is large, leaving only the tender leaves, and do not shred the radicchio until just before throwing it in your skillet because it can very quickly lose its texture.

Mushroom and Potato Stew

Serves 6
Prep time: 10 minutes / Cook time: 40 minutes
Worth the Wait

Sit back and relax with a comforting stew. Mushrooms add a pleasant earthiness and bone-boosting vitamin D. With bits of potato throughout, you'll get a starchy satisfaction—and potassium, too. This recipe is also ideal for meal planning: Prep it ahead or store any leftovers in mason jars. This soup defrosts and reheats well, holding up just like it did on the first day you made it.

2 tablespoons
    extra-virgin olive oil
5 ounces white
    mushrooms, sliced
½ cup diced carrots
½ cup diced
    yellow onion
½ cup diced celery
2½ cups low-sodium
    vegetable broth
1 cup diced tomatoes
1 teaspoon garlic
    powder
1 bay leaf
1 russet potato, peeled
    and finely diced
1 cup cooked chickpeas
Salt
Freshly ground black
    pepper
½ cup crumbled feta,
    for serving

1. In a large sauté pan or skillet, heat the olive oil over medium heat. Add the mushrooms and cook for 5 minutes, until they reduce in size and soften.

2. Add the carrots, onion, and celery to the pan and cook for 10 minutes, or until the onions are golden. Add the vegetable broth, tomatoes, garlic powder, and bay leaf and bring to a simmer. Add the potato.

3. Mix well and cover. Cook for 20 minutes or until the potato is fork-tender.

4. Add the chickpeas, stir, and remove the bay leaf. Season with salt and pepper. Serve, topped with feta, and enjoy!

5. Refrigerate in an airtight container for up 4 days.

PREP TIP: Be sure to taste the soup as you're seasoning it so that you don't over- or under-season. You can also experiment and add your favorite spices to make this dish your own.

Per serving: Calories: 169; Total Fat: 8g; Saturated Fat: 3g; Cholesterol: 11mg; Sodium: 136mg; Potassium: 463mg; Magnesium: 33mg; Carbohydrates: 19g; Sugars: 5g; Fiber: 4g; Protein: 6g; Added Sugars: 0g; Vitamin K: 11mcg

Barley Risotto with Sweet Potato and Spinach

VEGETARIAN
1 POT MEAL

Serves 4
Prep time: 10 minutes, plus soaking time / Cook time: 40 minutes

Barley is a nutty, chewy grain with a taste and texture that holds up well to earthy spinach, sweet potato, and a healthy amount of garlic. Sweet potato is rich in vitamin A, making it ideal for skin health.

2 tablespoons
extra-virgin olive oil,
divided

½ sweet onion, finely
chopped

1 teaspoon minced
garlic

1 cup pearl barley,
soaked overnight,
drained, and rinsed

2 sweet potatoes,
peeled and cut into
¼-inch pieces

3 cups low-sodium
vegetable stock

2 cups packed baby
spinach

½ cup grated
Parmesan cheese

Salt

Freshly ground black
pepper

1. Preheat the oven to 400°F.

2. In a large oven-safe skillet, heat 1 tablespoon of olive oil over medium-high heat. Sauté the onion and garlic until softened, about 3 minutes.

3. Stir in the barley, sweet potatoes, and vegetable stock. Cover the skillet and transfer it to the oven. Bake until the barley is tender and the liquid is absorbed, about 35 minutes.

4. Remove the skillet from the oven, stir in the spinach and Parmesan cheese, and drizzle on the remaining 1 tablespoon of olive oil. Season with salt and pepper and serve.

5. Refrigerate the leftovers in an airtight container for up to 5 days.

PREP TIP: Since you'll be soaking the barley overnight, it's also a good idea to peel and chop the sweet potato the night before you make this dish. Just store and refrigerate the sweet potato chunks in an airtight container until you're ready to use them. Meal prep can save you time and energy when you are ready to start cooking.

Per serving: Calories: 354; Total Fat: 11g; Saturated Fat: 3g; Cholesterol: 11mg; Sodium: 317mg; Potassium: 488mg; Magnesium: 73mg; Carbohydrates: 56g; Sugars: 4g; Fiber: 10g; Protein: 10g; Added Sugars: 0g; Vitamin K: 79mcg

Quinoa and Goat Cheese–Stuffed Sweet Potato

VEGETARIAN

Serves 4
Prep time: 15 minutes / Cook time: 1 hour
5 or Fewer Ingredients
Worth the Wait

Looking for ways to pack in the fiber? It doesn't get any easier than this recipe. A medium sweet potato contains 4 grams of fiber, and the quinoa adds more dietary fiber to the mix. But let's not forget about taste. The natural sweetness of the sweet potato paired with the creamy goat cheese is a match made in heaven.

4 sweet potatoes
Salt
Freshly ground black pepper
¾ cup quinoa, rinsed
½ cup crumbled goat cheese
2 tablespoons honey
2 tablespoons chopped fresh rosemary

1. Preheat the oven to 400°F. Line a baking sheet with aluminum foil or parchment paper.

2. Pierce the sweet potatoes a few times with a fork. Season with salt and pepper. Transfer to the prepared baking sheet and bake for 30 to 45 minutes, or until the sweet potatoes are semisoft.

3. While the sweet potatoes are in the oven, cook the quinoa according to the package instructions.

4. In a medium mixing bowl, combine the goat cheese, honey, and rosemary, and season with salt and pepper.

5. Once the quinoa is done cooking, fold it into the goat cheese mixture.

6. Remove the sweet potatoes from the oven, but leave the oven on. When the sweet potatoes are cool enough, carefully cut each one open lengthwise. Scoop out a divot in each sweet potato and stuff it with the quinoa and goat cheese mixture. Place the sweet potatoes back in the oven at 400°F for 10 to 15 minutes more, or until the cheese is gooey, golden, and slightly melted.

7. Refrigerate the leftovers in an airtight container for 3 to 5 days.

PREP TIP: I like to make large amounts of quinoa on a weekly basis and use it in recipes throughout the week. Once it's cooked, you can throw it in soups, use it in a stir-fry, or toss it in a salad. Quinoa typically doubles in amount when cooked, so when I plan on using it for the week, I make 2½ cups dried to get 5 cups cooked.

Per serving: Calories: 300; Total Fat: 5g; Saturated Fat: 2g; Cholesterol: 7mg; Sodium: 178mg; Potassium: 623mg; Magnesium: 99mg; Carbohydrates: 55g; Sugars: 5g; Fiber: 6g; Protein: 9g; Added Sugars: 9g; Vitamin K: 3mcg

Lentil Ragout

Serves 6
Prep time: 15 minutes / Cook time: 50 minutes
Worth the Wait

A ragout is essentially a French variation of a stew. Although usually made with meat and vegetables, this tasty version is made with lentils, which are low in calories, rich in iron and folate, and an excellent source of protein. Serve this with garlic bread for wiping the bowl clean, or use it as a hearty meat-sauce alternative over your favorite noodles.

¼ cup extra-virgin olive oil

1 onion, finely chopped

4 carrots, peeled and cut into ¼-inch dice

2 celery stalks, cut into ¼-inch-thick slices

4 garlic cloves, mashed

1 pound dried French green lentils, rinsed and picked over for debris

4 thyme sprigs

2 bay leaves

½ teaspoon dried oregano

½ teaspoon cayenne pepper

⅛ teaspoon salt

1. In a heavy-bottomed pot, heat the olive oil over medium heat.

2. Add the onion and cook for 5 minutes.

3. Add the carrots, celery, and garlic and cook, stirring often, for 10 minutes more.

4. Stir in the lentils, thyme, bay leaves, oregano, cayenne, salt, black pepper, broth, and water. Increase the heat to medium-high and bring the mixture to a boil. Reduce the heat to medium-low and cook, uncovered, for 30 minutes or until the lentils are tender.

5. Remove and discard the thyme and bay leaves. Stir in the vinegar and serve.

Ingredients continued on page 91

⅛ teaspoon freshly
ground black pepper
2 cups vegetable broth
2 cups water
2 tablespoons red wine
vinegar

6. Refrigerate the leftovers in an airtight container for up to 3 days. If prepping in advance, cool completely before storing.

PREP TIP: Low-sodium broths can be unpredictable in flavor (and often don't taste so great). To maintain a good balance of flavor while keeping the sodium content in check, in this recipe we use a ratio of ½ water to ½ vegetable broth for the liquid.

SUBSTITUTION TIP: Use 1 cup of pearl onions, 4 baby zucchini (halved), and 8 ounces of baby carrots instead of the large vegetables.

Per serving: Calories: 375; Total Fat: 10g; Saturated Fat: 1g; Cholesterol: 0mg; Sodium: 91mg; Potassium: 698mg; Magnesium: 44mg; Carbohydrates: 54g; Sugars: 4g; Fiber: 10g; Protein: 19g; Added Sugars: 0g; Vitamin K: 17mcg

Eggplant and Rice Casserole

Serves 4
Prep time: 30 minutes / Cook time: 40 minutes
Worth the Wait

Eggplant is a good source of fiber and blood pressure–regulating potassium. It's also a source of anthocyanins, antioxidants responsible for the eggplant's rich, vibrant color. The spices, onion, and garlic in this recipe are heated to maximal flavor and there is no added salt, making this dish a delicious low-sodium meal.

FOR THE SAUCE

⅓ cup extra-virgin
   olive oil
1 small onion, chopped
4 garlic cloves, mashed
6 ripe tomatoes,
   peeled and chopped
2 tablespoons
   tomato paste
1 teaspoon dried
   oregano
¼ teaspoon ground
   nutmeg
¼ teaspoon
   ground cumin

TO MAKE THE SAUCE

1. In a heavy-bottomed saucepan, heat the olive oil over medium heat. Add the onion and cook for 5 minutes.

2. Stir in the garlic, tomatoes, tomato paste, oregano, nutmeg, and cumin. Bring to a boil. Cover, reduce the heat to low, and simmer for 10 minutes. Remove from the heat and set aside.

TO MAKE THE CASSEROLE

3. Preheat the broiler.

4. While the sauce simmers, drizzle the eggplants with the olive oil and place them on a baking sheet. Broil for about 5 minutes, until golden. Remove and let cool.

5. Turn the oven to 375°F. Arrange the cooled eggplants, cut-side up, in a 9 x 13-inch baking dish. Gently scoop out some flesh to make room for the stuffing.

Ingredients continued on page 93

FOR THE CASSEROLE

4 (6-inch) Japanese eggplants, halved lengthwise

2 tablespoons extra-virgin olive oil

1 cup cooked rice

2 tablespoons pine nuts, toasted

1 cup water

6. In a bowl, combine half the tomato sauce, the cooked rice, and pine nuts. Fill each eggplant half with the rice mixture.

7. In the same bowl, combine the remaining half of the tomato sauce and the water. Pour over the eggplant.

8. Bake, covered, for 20 minutes until the eggplant is soft.

9. Store the leftovers in an airtight container for 3 to 5 days.

Per serving: Calories: 487; Total Fat: 29g; Saturated Fat: 4g; Cholesterol: 0mg; Sodium: 27mg; Potassium: 1856mg; Magnesium: 120mg; Carbohydrates: 55g; Sugars: 26g; Fiber: 20g; Protein: 9g; Added Sugars: 0g; Vitamin K: 53mcg

Vegetable Paella

Serves 6
Prep time: 25 minutes / Cook time: 45 minutes
Worth the Wait

Paella originated in Valencia, a port city on the southeastern coast of Spain. And this beautiful dish gets its name from the pan it's cooked in. If you don't have a paella pan; any large oven-safe skillet with deep sides will work.

¼ cup extra-virgin olive oil

1 large sweet onion, chopped

1 large red bell pepper, seeded and chopped

1 large green bell pepper, seeded and chopped

3 garlic cloves, finely minced

1 teaspoon smoked paprika

5 saffron threads (see substitution tip)

1 zucchini, cut into ½-inch cubes

4 large ripe tomatoes, peeled, seeded, and chopped

1½ cups short-grain rice

3 cups vegetable broth, warmed

1. Preheat the oven to 350°F.

2. In a paella pan or large oven-safe skillet, heat the olive oil over medium heat.

3. Add the onion and red and green bell peppers and cook for 10 minutes.

4. Stir in the garlic, paprika, saffron, zucchini, and tomatoes. Turn the heat to medium-low and cook for 10 minutes.

5. Stir in the rice and vegetable broth. Increase the heat to medium-high to bring the paella to a boil. Reduce the heat to medium-low and cook for 15 minutes. Cover the pan with aluminum foil and put it in the oven.

6. Bake for 10 minutes or until the broth is absorbed.

7. Refrigerate the leftovers in an airtight container for 3 to 5 days.

SUBSTITUTION TIP: Skip the saffron and use ¼ teaspoon of ground turmeric instead to get the lovely yellow hue of traditional paella.

Per serving: Calories: 313; Total Fat: 10g; Saturated Fat: 1g; Cholesterol: 0mg; Sodium: 13mg; Potassium: 568mg; Magnesium: 40mg; Carbohydrates: 51g; Sugars: 7g; Fiber: 5g; Protein: 6g; Added Sugars: 0g; Vitamin K: 20mcg

Butternut Squash, Zucchini, and Bulgur Pilaf

DAIRY-FREE
VEGETARIAN

Serves 4
Prep time: 25 minutes / Cook time: 50 minutes
Worth the Wait

This potassium-rich dish delights with the creaminess of the butternut squash, a great complement to the chewiness of the bulgur, the crunch of the walnuts, and the zesty jalapeño kick.

3 pounds butternut squash, peeled, seeded, and cut into ½-inch-thick half-moons

4 tablespoons extra-virgin olive oil, divided

1 small onion, finely chopped

4 scallions, white and green parts, chopped

1 zucchini, diced

1 jalapeño pepper, seeded and finely chopped

½ red bell pepper, chopped

2 tomatoes, diced

¼ cup chopped fresh cilantro

½ cup coarse bulgur

¼ cup coarsely chopped walnuts

1. Preheat the oven to 400°F.

2. On a baking sheet, toss together the butternut squash and 1 tablespoon of the olive oil until coated. Spread into a single layer. Bake for 10 minutes. Remove from the oven and set aside.

3. In a large skillet, heat the remaining 3 tablespoons of olive oil over medium heat.

4. Add the onion and cook for 5 minutes. Add the scallions, zucchini, jalapeño, red bell pepper, tomatoes, and cilantro. Toss to coat. Reduce the heat to medium-low and cook for 10 minutes.

5. Stir in the bulgur and bring the mixture to a boil. Reduce the heat to low, cover the skillet, and cook for 15 minutes.

6. Remove the skillet from the heat, stir in the butternut squash and walnuts, cover, and let the pilaf rest for 10 minutes before serving.

7. Refrigerate the leftovers in an airtight container for 2 days.

Per serving: Calories: 366; Total Fat: 19g; Saturated Fat: 2g; Cholesterol: 0mg; Sodium: 24mg; Potassium: 1288mg; Magnesium: 140mg; Carbohydrates: 49g; Sugars: 10g; Fiber: 10g; Protein: 7g; Added Sugars: 0g; Vitamin K: 54mcg

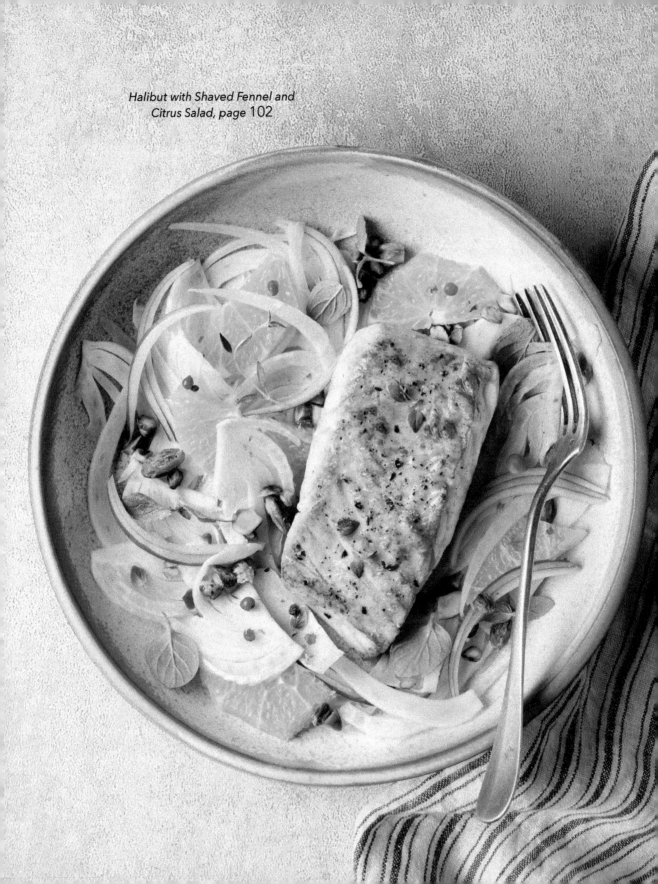

*Halibut with Shaved Fennel and
Citrus Salad, page 102*

Fish and Seafood

Citrus-Herb Scallops

Serves 4
Prep time: 10 minutes / Cook time: 5 minutes
5 or Fewer Ingredients

Scallops are best eaten fresh, which means enjoying them between October and March, although you can get outstanding-quality frozen products. Scallops are often considered unhealthy because they are often served with high-calorie, fat-laden sauces, but this simple, fresh preparation allows the scallops to shine through. Scallops are a great source of protein, potassium, and magnesium.

1 pound sea scallops
Salt
Freshly ground black pepper
2 tablespoons extra-virgin olive oil
Juice of 1 lime
Pinch red pepper flakes
1 tablespoon chopped fresh cilantro

1. Season the scallops lightly with salt and black pepper.

2. In a large skillet, heat the olive oil over medium-high heat. Add the scallops to the skillet, making sure they do not touch one another.

3. Sear on both sides, turning once, for a total of about 3 minutes. Add the lime juice and red pepper flakes to the skillet and toss the scallops in the juice. Serve topped with cilantro.

4. Scallops are best enjoyed right away. If you have any leftovers, refrigerate them in an airtight container for up to 2 days.

PREP TIP: Fresh scallops are in season from late fall through winter, so that is the best time to make this special dish. Look for drier scallops, not stored in a milky liquid called sodium triphosphate. This additive causes the scallops to soak up water, which means you are paying for water weight and your scallops will have less flavor.

Per serving: Calories: 141; Total Fat: 7g; Saturated Fat: 1g; Cholesterol: 27mg; Sodium: 484mg; Potassium: 247mg; Magnesium: 26mg; Carbohydrates: 5g; Sugars: 0g; Fiber: 0g; Protein: 14g; Added Sugars: 0g; Vitamin K: 5mcg

Trout with Ruby Red Grapefruit Relish

DAIRY-FREE

Serves 4
Prep time: 15 minutes / Cook time: 15 minutes

It is no surprise that seafood plays such a huge role in the Italian diet when you consider that almost every region in Italy has a coastline stretch on the Mediterranean, providing heaps of seafood and wonderful freshwater fish like trout. In this recipe, pepperoncini add a potent heat to the tart, colorful relish, and they contain even more vitamin C than the citrus fruit, as well as vitamins A and B, fiber, and potassium.

1 ruby red grapefruit, peeled, sectioned, and chopped
1 large navel orange, peeled, sectioned, and chopped
¼ English cucumber, chopped
2 tablespoons chopped red onion
1 tablespoon grated lime zest
1 teaspoon minced fresh or canned pepperoncini
1 teaspoon chopped fresh thyme
4 (4-ounce) trout fillets
Salt
Freshly ground black pepper
1 tablespoon extra-virgin olive oil

1. Preheat the oven to 400°F.

2. In a medium bowl, stir together the grapefruit, orange, cucumber, onion, lime zest, pepperoncini, and thyme. Cover the relish with plastic wrap and set it aside in the refrigerator.

3. Season the trout lightly with salt and pepper and place it on a baking sheet.

4. Brush the fish with olive oil and roast it in the oven until it flakes easily with a fork, about 15 minutes. Serve topped with the chilled relish.

5. Refrigerate the leftovers in an airtight container for 3 to 4 days.

SUBSTITUTION TIP: You can easily swap out the large navel orange for 6 to 8 clementines. The benefit of those little mandarin oranges is that they are easy to peel, contain less of the bitter white pith, and have small segments, so they will require less fuss and less chopping.

Per serving: Calories: 237; Total Fat: 10g; Saturated Fat: 2g; Cholesterol: 67mg; Sodium: 97mg; Potassium: 636mg; Magnesium: 41mg; Carbohydrates: 12g; Sugars: 9g; Fiber: 2g; Protein: 24g; Added Sugars: 0g; Vitamin K: 5mcg

Mussels in Ginger-Garlic Broth

Serves 4
Prep time: 5 minutes / Cook time: 15 minutes

When purchasing ingredients for and preparing this dish, check that your mussels aren't cracked or discolored. They should have a sweet, salty scent. Serve it with steamed broccoli and a ¼-inch slice of French baguette to soak up the broth.

**2 tablespoons
extra-virgin olive oil**
**½ sweet onion, finely
chopped**
**1 tablespoon plus
1 teaspoon minced
garlic plus 1 teaspoon**
**1 teaspoon grated
fresh ginger**
Pinch salt
¼ teaspoon turmeric
**1 teaspoon Italian
seasoning**
**½ cup white wine
(Chardonnay works
well)**
½ cup water
**Grated zest and juice
of 1 Meyer lemon,
divided**
**1½ pounds fresh
mussels, scrubbed
and debearded (or
frozen, thawed)**
**2 tablespoons finely
chopped cilantro**

1. In a large skillet, heat the olive oil over medium-high heat and sauté the onion, garlic, and ginger until softened, about 3 minutes.

2. Add the salt, turmeric, and Italian seasoning to the skillet and stir to combine.

3. Stir in the white wine, water, lemon zest, and 1 tablespoon of the lemon juice.

4. Add the mussels, cover, and steam until the shells are open, about 8 minutes. Remove any unopened shells and take the skillet off the heat.

5. Stir in the cilantro and the remaining lemon juice, and serve.

6. Refrigerate the leftovers in a shallow, airtight container for 3 to 4 days.

PREP TIP: To add a bit more tang, add ¼ teaspoon of Dijon mustard in step 3. Trust me, it's good!

Per serving: Calories: 134; Total Fat: 8g; Saturated Fat: 1g; Cholesterol: 12mg; Sodium: 163mg; Potassium: 210mg; Magnesium: 21mg; Carbohydrates: 6g; Sugars: 1g; Fiber: 0g; Protein: 5g; Added Sugars: 0g; Vitamin K: 6mcg

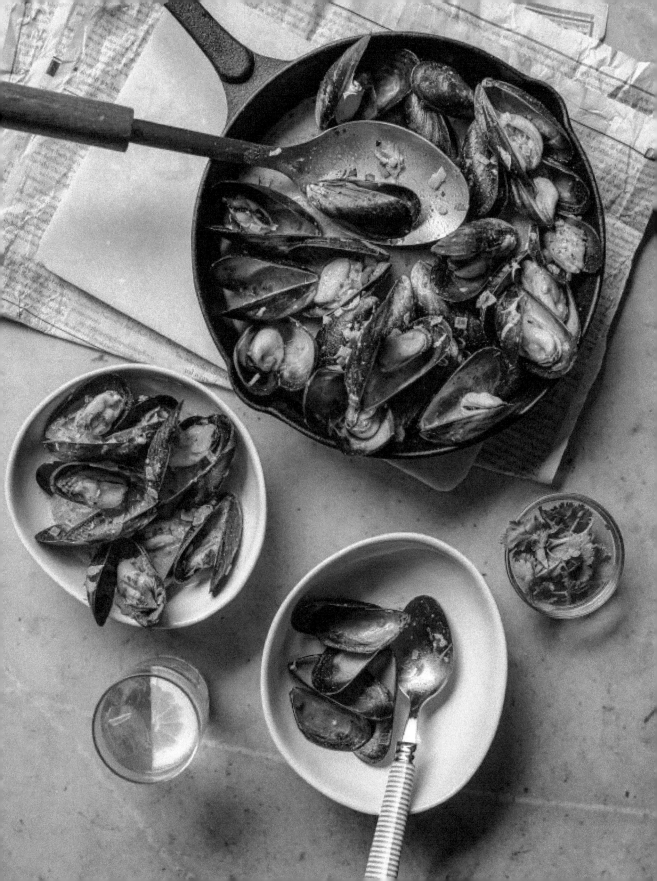

Halibut with Shaved Fennel and Citrus Salad

DAIRY-FREE
QUICK

Serves 4
Prep time: 10 minutes / Cook time: 15 minutes

The bulb of the fennel plant has a very mild licorice taste that even people who don't like licorice will enjoy. Fennel also offers a crisp texture that is perfect when it is eaten raw or sautéed. Serve this delightful halibut entrée over a bed of leafy greens or with a side of green beans for some more plant-based goodness.

3 tablespoons extra-virgin olive oil, divided

3 tablespoons sherry vinegar

2 teaspoons honey

Juice of 1 lemon

2 tablespoons grated orange zest, plus 2 oranges, peeled and sliced

2 bulbs fennel, cored and thinly shaved

¼ cup fresh mint, plus 2 tablespoons

Kosher salt

Freshly ground black pepper

1. To make the dressing, whisk together 1 tablespoon of the olive oil, the vinegar, honey, lemon juice, and orange zest.

2. Put the shaved fennel and ¼ cup of the mint in a large bowl and drizzle it with the dressing. Season with salt and pepper. Add the orange slices and toss. Sprinkle the salad with the pistachios. Set aside.

3. Pat the fish dry with a paper towel and season both sides with salt and pepper. In a large skillet, heat the remaining 2 tablespoons of olive oil over medium-high heat. Add the garlic and shallot. Cook for 1 to 2 minutes, until fragrant. Add the thyme and halibut fillets. Cook for 3 to 4 minutes, then flip the fillets. Cook the other side for 4 to 5 minutes more, until the fish is opaque and flakes with a fork.

Ingredients continued on page 103

¼ cup unsalted
pistachios, roughly
chopped
4 (4-ounce) halibut fillets
1 clove garlic, sliced
1 shallot, sliced
2 thyme leaves and
sprigs

4. To serve, transfer the fennel salad to a serving
dish and place the halibut on top. Garnish with
the remaining 2 tablespoons of mint and enjoy.

5. Refrigerate the leftovers in an airtight container for
3 to 4 days.

SUBSTITUTION TIP: Halibut is a mild whitefish and has a
similar taste, texture, and appearance to cod. You can use
the two types of fish in recipes interchangeably and just
buy what is cheaper or more convenient.

Per serving: Calories: 329; Total Fat: 16g; Saturated Fat: 2g;
Cholesterol: 56mg; Sodium: 182mg; Potassium: 1244mg;
Magnesium: 70mg; Carbohydrates: 24g; Sugars: 11g; Fiber: 7g;
Protein: 25g; Added Sugars: 3g; Vitamin K: 80mcg

Tuna Couscous Sauté

Serves 4
Prep time: 15 minutes / Cook time: 10 minutes
5 or Fewer Ingredients

Couscous, a staple of North African cooking, is a pasta (not a grain) that is unbelievably easy to prepare. Nutritionally, couscous provides 6 grams of protein per one cup cooked, and it has some calcium and fiber, too. This dish complements the mild and chewy couscous with an array of sautéed vegetables—a combo that pairs nicely with the tuna. A nice fruit salad would be the perfect finish to this light meal.

1 cup dry couscous
2 tablespoons extra-virgin olive oil
2 large carrots, thinly sliced
4 cups green beans, cut into 1-inch pieces
2 yellow zucchini, sliced in half lengthwise and cut into half-moons
Salt
Freshly ground black pepper
2 (4-ounce) cans chunk albacore tuna

Per serving: Calories: 348; Total Fat: 9g; Saturated Fat: 2g; Cholesterol: 21mg; Sodium: 269mg; Potassium: 771mg; Magnesium: 82mg; Carbohydrates: 47g; Sugars: 7g; Fiber: 7g; Protein: 20g; Added Sugars: 0g; Vitamin K: 29mcg

1. Prepare the couscous according to package directions and set it aside.

2. In a large skillet, heat the olive oil over medium-high heat.

3. Sauté the carrots until tender-crisp, about 5 minutes.

4. Add the green beans and zucchini and sauté until the vegetables are tender, about 5 minutes.

5. Season the vegetables with salt and pepper.

6. Spoon the couscous into four bowls and evenly divide the vegetables among them.

7. Serve the couscous topped with the tuna.

8. Refrigerate the leftovers in an airtight container for 3 to 4 days.

PREP TIP: There are several varieties of couscous to choose from for this dish. The best type, which can be difficult to find, is Israeli couscous, which has larger pea-size granules. It's usually made of semolina and whole wheat and is toasted rather than dried like regular couscous. This means the flavor is richer and nuttier.

Sun-Dried Tomato Pesto Snapper

Serves 4
Prep time: 5 minutes / Cook time: 15 minutes
5 or Fewer Ingredients

Sun-dried tomato pesto adds a vibrant color and tangy, rich flavor to plenty of things. You may envision this brightly colored condiment in a pasta or as a topping for a crusty bread appetizer or grilled asparagus spears, but liberally spreading this pesto on fish is another quick way to make an outstanding meal. Regular basil pesto would be excellent, too, if you prefer that flavor profile.

1 sweet onion, cut into ¼-inch slices

4 (5-ounce) snapper fillets

Freshly ground black pepper

4 tablespoons sun-dried tomato pesto

2 tablespoons finely chopped fresh basil

Per serving: Calories: 221; Total Fat: 9g; Saturated Fat: 1g; Cholesterol: 52mg; Sodium: 100mg; Potassium: 751mg; Magnesium: 56mg; Carbohydrates: 4g; Sugars: 2g; Fiber: 1g; Protein: 29g; Added Sugars: 0g; Vitamin K: 11mcg

1. Preheat the oven to 400°F. Line a baking dish with parchment paper and arrange the onion slices on the parchment.

2. Pat the snapper fillets dry with a paper towel and season them lightly with pepper.

3. Place the fillets on the onions and spread 1 tablespoon of pesto on each fillet.

4. Bake until the fish flakes easily with a fork, 12 to 15 minutes.

5. Serve topped with the basil.

6. Refrigerate the leftovers in an airtight container for 2 to 3 days.

PREP TIP: Sun-dried tomato pesto is a simple product to whip up in your kitchen if you have a blender or food processor. Pulse 1 cup of sun-dried tomatoes, ½ cup of basil, ¼ cup of Parmesan cheese, ¼ cup of olive oil, and 4 garlic cloves until a thick paste forms. Store the pesto in the refrigerator for up to 1 week in a sealed container.

Baked Spanish Salmon

DAIRY-FREE

Serves 4
Prep time: 10 minutes / Cook time: 20 minutes

Looking for a unique way to enjoy omega-3-rich salmon? This dish has got two intense flavor notes that make it absolutely appealing. The sweet taste of the red onion and carrots is perfectly balanced by the sharp flavor of the fennel and stuffed olives.

2 small red onions, thinly sliced

1 cup shaved fennel bulb

1 cup cherry tomatoes

15 green pimento olives

Salt

Freshly ground black pepper

1 teaspoon cumin seeds

½ teaspoon smoked paprika

4 (8-ounce) salmon fillets

½ cup vegetable broth

2 to 4 tablespoons extra-virgin olive oil, for drizzling

2 cups cooked couscous

1. Put the oven racks in the middle of the oven and preheat the oven to 375°F.

2. On two baking sheets, spread out the onions, fennel, tomatoes, and olives. Season them with the salt, pepper, cumin, and paprika.

3. Place the fish over the vegetables, season them with salt, and gently pour the broth over the two baking sheets. Drizzle a light stream of olive oil over the baking sheets before popping them in the oven.

4. Bake the vegetables and fish for 20 minutes, checking halfway through to ensure nothing is burning. Serve the vegetables and fish over the couscous.

5. Refrigerate the leftovers in an airtight container for 3 to 4 days.

SUBSTITUTION TIP: If salmon isn't available, try your next favorite hearty fish, like swordfish.

Per serving: Calories: 515; Total Fat: 23g; Saturated Fat: 3g; Cholesterol: 125mg; Sodium: 316mg; Potassium: 1407mg; Magnesium: 87mg; Carbohydrates: 25g; Sugars: 3g; Fiber: 3g; Protein: 49g; Added Sugars: 0g; Vitamin K: 21mcg

Sole en Papillote

Serves 4
Prep time: 10 minutes / Cook time: 15 minutes

This simple fish en papillote—also known as fish in parchment—is just as easy to cook as it is to clean up! The fish is steamed in parchment paper, allowing the lemon and herbs to infuse the fish and bok choy with their delicious flavors.

4 (4-ounce) sole fillets
Kosher salt
Freshly ground black pepper
2 shallots, diced
1 tablespoon capers
4 heads baby bok choy
4 garlic cloves, smashed
4 thyme sprigs
1 tablespoon extra-virgin olive oil
1 lemon, thinly sliced

Per serving: Calories: 132; Total Fat: 6g; Saturated Fat: 1g; Cholesterol: 51mg; Sodium: 434mg; Potassium: 299mg; Magnesium: 29mg; Carbohydrates: 5g; Sugars: 2g; Fiber: 1g; Protein: 15g; Added Sugars: 0g; Vitamin K: 37mcg

1. Preheat the oven to 400°F.

2. Pat the fish dry with a paper towel. Fold four pieces of parchment paper in half and open them back up. Place 1 fillet on one half of each piece of parchment paper. Season both sides of each fillet with salt and black pepper.

3. Divide the shallots and capers among the fillets. Then place 1 head of bok choy, 1 smashed garlic clove, and 1 thyme sprig on top of each fillet. Brush with the olive oil and top with the lemon slices.

4. Fold the other side of the parchment over and crimp the edges tightly closed. Place the packages on a large rimmed baking sheet.

5. Bake for 10 to 12 minutes. Once done baking, carefully (the steam will be hot!) cut the pouches open. Serve warm.

6. Refrigerate the leftovers in an airtight container for up to 2 days.

PREP TIP: Make sure you cut the parchment paper big enough to cover the entire fillet. It's always better to have a piece that is too big rather than too small. If you don't have parchment, aluminum foil will work as well.

Pistachio-Encrusted Scallops

DAIRY-FREE
QUICK

Serves 4
Prep time: 15 minutes / Cook time: 5 minutes
5 or Fewer Ingredients

Scallops look intimidating but are easy and quick to prepare and do not need many added ingredients to become a restaurant-quality meal. Extra-virgin olive oil is the fat of choice for this dish for its omega-3 content and because it is lower in saturated fat than butter. To make this a meal, serve the scallops with grilled asparagus and a side of couscous.

1 pound sea scallops, cleaned
⅛ teaspoon salt, for seasoning
Freshly ground black pepper
1 cup crushed, roasted, unsalted pistachios
4 tablespoons extra-virgin olive oil, divided
Juice of 1 lime

Per serving: Calories: 373; Total Fat: 28g; Saturated Fat: 4g; Cholesterol: 27mg; Sodium: 523mg; Potassium: 561mg; Magnesium: 63mg; Carbohydrates: 13g; Sugars: 3g; Fiber: 3g; Protein: 20g; Added Sugars: 0g; Vitamin K: 30mcg

1. Pat the scallops dry with a paper towel and season them lightly on all sides with salt and pepper.

2. Place the pistachios in a large bowl and dredge the scallops in the crushed nuts, making sure to coat all sides.

3. In a large skillet, heat 2 tablespoons of the olive oil over high heat.

4. Sear the scallops until they are golden brown, about 2 minutes, and then turn them over.

5. Add the remaining 2 tablespoons of olive oil to the skillet, so the scallops don't dry out, and continue cooking the scallops for 3 minutes more.

6. Serve immediately with a squeeze of lime juice.

7. Scallops are best enjoyed right away, but you can refrigerate the leftovers in an airtight container for up to 2 days.

SUBSTITUTION TIP: Other nut crusts made from almonds, pecans, macadamia nuts, and hazelnuts will work just as well with these golden scallops. Use 1 cup of the crushed nut of your choice and follow the recipe directions.

Pan-Seared Shrimp Skewers

Serves 4
Prep time: 20 minutes / Cook time: 10 minutes
5 or Fewer Ingredients

Searching for a simple lemon shrimp recipe that goes perfectly over pasta or rice? Look no further than this speedy dish. You can also serve the tender pink shrimp skewers with baked potatoes or your favorite sautéed vegetables.

¼ cup extra-virgin
   olive oil
Grated zest and juice
   of 1 lemon, divided
1 tablespoon dried
   oregano
¼ teaspoon red pepper
   flakes (optional)
Salt
Freshly ground black
   pepper
1 pound medium
   shrimp (36/40 count),
   peeled and deveined

1. In a large bowl, stir together the olive oil, lemon zest, oregano, and red pepper flakes (if using). Season with salt and black pepper. Add the shrimp and mix well. Cover the bowl with plastic wrap and refrigerate for 15 minutes.

2. Remove the bowl from the refrigerator and thread the shrimp onto skewers. Discard any remaining marinade.

3. Heat a large skillet over medium heat. Place the skewers in the skillet and sear the shrimp for 3 to 4 minutes per side, until just cooked through.

4. Drizzle with the lemon juice and serve.

5. Refrigerate in an airtight container for up to 2 days.

PREP TIP: Top a lovely pilaf or couscous dish with a couple of these skewers for a light meal.

Per serving: Calories: 145; Total Fat: 8g; Saturated Fat: 1g; Cholesterol: 143mg; Sodium: 681mg; Potassium: 150mg; Magnesium: 28mg; Carbohydrates: 2g; Sugars: 0g; Fiber: 0g; Protein: 15g; Added Sugars: 0g; Vitamin K: 9mcg

Mediterranean Salmon Wraps

QUICK

Serves 4
Prep time: 10 minutes

This simple recipe is perfect for pack-and-go lunches or quick dinners on busy weeknights. You can use the same salmon mix to build sandwiches, lettuce wraps, and salads when you aren't in the mood for a tortilla wrap. And the leftovers taste even better once the flavors have a chance to mingle.

2 (6-ounce) cans salmon, drained
¼ cup chopped fresh parsley
¼ cup pitted, chopped Kalamata olives
¼ cup diced red onion
1 tablespoon extra-virgin olive oil
½ teaspoon grated lemon zest and juice of 1 lemon
⅛ teaspoon kosher salt
2 cups chopped romaine
4 small (6-inch) whole-wheat tortillas
½ cup diced red bell pepper
1 Roma tomato, thinly sliced
½ cup crumbled feta cheese

1. In a large bowl, combine the salmon, parsley, olives, onion, olive oil, and lemon zest and juice. Season with the salt, and stir to combine.

2. Layer ½ cup of the chopped romaine in the center of each tortilla. Top each tortilla with a quarter each of the salmon mixture and bell peppers, and two slices of tomato. Sprinkle with the feta cheese.

3. Fold in each tortilla about 1 inch from the end of the filling on each side. Tightly roll, being careful not to break the wrap. Secure the edge of the wrap underneath; then cut in half. Serve immediately.

4. It's best to consume the full wrap on the day you plan to serve it. Refrigerate the leftovers in an airtight container for up to 24 hours.

PREP TIP: If prepping for lunches, make the salmon mix and prepare the veggies but don't roll the wraps until you're ready to serve the meal. This will help you avoid an overly soggy wrap that tears or breaks open.

Per serving: Calories: 334; Total Fat: 16g; Saturated Fat: 6g; Cholesterol: 76mg; Sodium: 758mg; Potassium: 538mg; Magnesium: 72mg; Carbohydrates: 25g; Sugars: 4g; Fiber: 6g; Protein: 24g; Added Sugars: 0g; Vitamin K: 92mcg

Baking Sheet Spicy Shrimp with Vegetables

Serves 4
Prep time: 15 minutes / Cook time: 15 minutes

Shrimp cooks very quickly, so it is a great choice when you need a nutritious meal in a hurry. The colorful assortment of vegetables in this recipe cooks in the same amount of time as the shellfish. Bok choy is not a traditional Mediterranean vegetable, but it shares the health benefits of the other members of the cabbage family and is mild enough to combine well with any ingredient.

1 pound shrimp, peeled and deveined

3 baby bok choy, quartered

10 asparagus spears, trimmed and halved

1 yellow zucchini, sliced

1 red bell pepper, cut into thin strips

1 sweet onion, thinly sliced

1 tablespoon extra-virgin olive oil

½ teaspoon smoked paprika

½ teaspoon chili powder

½ teaspoon garlic powder

½ teaspoon ground cumin

Juice of 1 lime

1. Preheat the oven to 400°F.

2. In a large bowl, toss together the shrimp, bok choy, asparagus, zucchini, bell pepper, onion, olive oil, paprika, chili powder, garlic powder, and cumin until the shrimp are well coated. Spread the shrimp and vegetables on a rimmed baking sheet.

3. Bake until the shrimp are cooked through and the vegetables are tender, stirring a few times, 10 to 12 minutes. Squeeze the lime juice over the shrimp and vegetables. Serve.

4. Refrigerate the leftovers in an airtight container for up to 2 days.

PREP TIP: To make this a one-pot meal and save time washing dishes, toss all the ingredients directly on the rimmed baking sheet using a pair of tongs.

Per serving: Calories: 183; Total Fat: 4g; Saturated Fat: 1g; Cholesterol: 183mg; Sodium: 161mg; Potassium: 743mg; Magnesium: 70 mg; Carbohydrates: 12g; Sugars: 6g; Fiber: 4g; Protein: 26g; Added Sugars: 0g; Vitamin K: 61mcg

Whole Baked Trout with Lemon and Herbs

DAIRY-FREE
QUICK

Serves 4
Prep time: 10 minutes / Cook time: 20 minutes
5 or Fewer Ingredients

Tender, fragrant baked whole fish festooned with herbs on serving platters in the middle of the table is a common sight in many North African and Mediterranean countries. Stuffing the cavity of the cleaned fish with herbs, vegetables, and citrus fruit is an effective way to infuse the fish with flavor.

3 teaspoons extra-virgin olive oil, divided
2 (8-ounce) whole trout, cleaned
Salt
Freshly ground black pepper
1 lemon, thinly sliced into about 6 pieces
1 tablespoon finely chopped fresh dill
1 tablespoon chopped fresh parsley
½ cup low-sodium fish stock

1. Preheat the oven to 400°F.

2. Lightly grease a 9 x 13-inch baking dish with 1 teaspoon of olive oil.

3. Rinse the trout, pat it dry with a paper towel, and coat it with the remaining 2 teaspoons of olive oil. Season with salt and pepper.

4. Stuff the interior of the trout with the lemon slices, dill, and parsley and place into the prepared baking dish. Bake the fish for 10 minutes; then add the fish stock to the dish.

5. Continue to bake until the fish flakes easily with a fork, about 10 minutes. Serve.

6. Refrigerate the leftovers in an airtight container for 3 to 4 days.

Per serving: Calories: 203; Total Fat: 11g; Saturated Fat: 2g; Cholesterol: 66mg; Sodium: 99mg; Potassium: 434mg; Magnesium: 30mg; Carbohydrates: 1g; Sugars: 0g; Fiber: 0g; Protein: 24g; Added Sugars: 0g; Vitamin K: 18mcg

PREP TIP: If you don't have fish stock on hand, you can swap it out for water. The advantage of stock is that it adds more flavor. But since this fish is already stuffed and full of citrus-herbal flavor and only a bit of stock is required, using water instead will be just fine. Want to punch it up? Add a pinch of pepper flakes, cumin, or smoked paprika to your final presentation.

Mediterranean Snapper with Olives and Feta

Serves 4
Prep time: 10 minutes / Cook time: 25 minutes

Snapper stands up well to strong, fragrant Mediterranean flavors like this recipe's olives and garlic. This dish will work well with a side of couscous or over a bed of greens.

3 tablespoons
  extra-virgin olive oil,
  divided, plus more for
  brushing
4 (4- or 5-ounce)
  snapper fillets
½ teaspoon salt
¼ teaspoon black
  pepper
1 onion, chopped
2 garlic cloves, minced
1 teaspoon dried
  oregano
1 (14.5-ounce) can
  diced tomatoes
½ cup chopped pitted
  Kalamata olives
¼ cup crumbled feta
  cheese
2 tablespoons chopped
  fresh flat-leaf parsley

Per serving: Calories: 307; Total Fat: 16g; Saturated Fat: 3g; Cholesterol: 61mg; Sodium: 719mg; Potassium: 866mg; Magnesium: 63mg; Carbohydrates: 9g; Sugars: 4g; Fiber: 3g; Protein: 32g; Added Sugars: 0g; Vitamin K: 42mcg

1. Preheat the oven to 425°F. Brush a 3-quart (9 x 13-inch) baking dish lightly with olive oil.

2. Place the snapper in the prepared baking dish. Massage it gently with 2 tablespoons of olive oil; then season with the salt and pepper.

3. In a large skillet, heat the remaining 1 tablespoon of olive oil over medium heat. Add the onion, garlic, and oregano and cook for about 3 minutes, until the onion starts to soften.

4. Add the tomatoes and their juices and the olives and cook for 5 minutes to warm through and combine the flavors.

5. Spoon the tomato mixture over the fish.

6. Bake for 10 to 15 minutes, until the fish is tender and flakes easily with a fork.

7. Serve with a sprinkling of crumbled feta cheese and chopped parsley.

8. Refrigerate the leftovers in an airtight container for 3 to 4 days.

PREP TIP: Meal prep ahead of time by chopping your onion and garlic the night before you make this dish; chop your fresh herbs just a few hours before so they don't lose their fresh, vibrant flavor.

Moroccan Cod

DAIRY-FREE
1 POT MEAL

Serves 4
Prep time: 10 minutes / Cook time: 35 minutes

Cod is an excellent source of B-vitamins, omega-3s, and minerals including phosphorus and selenium. Phosphorus helps the body maintain and repair our cells, and selenium helps protect our DNA. This recipe uses Moroccan spices to complement the mildness of the cod and potatoes.

2 russet potatoes, peeled and cut into large chunks
6 carrots, cut into large chunks
4 tablespoons extra-virgin olive oil, divided
1½ teaspoons salt, divided
4 (6-ounce) cod fillets
½ teaspoon ground cumin
½ teaspoon paprika
¼ teaspoon ground turmeric
1 large red onion, cut into large chunks
Fresh flat-leaf parsley, chopped, for garnish

Per serving: Calories: 405; Total Fat: 15g; Saturated Fat: 2g; Cholesterol: 73mg; Sodium: 1046mg; Potassium: 1563mg; Magnesium: 98mg; Carbohydrates: 34g; Sugars: 7g; Fiber: 5g; Protein: 34g; Added Sugars: 0g; Vitamin K: 25mcg

1. Preheat the oven to 425°F. Line a rimmed baking sheet with aluminum foil.

2. Toss the potatoes and carrots on the prepared baking sheet with 3 tablespoons of olive oil and 1 teaspoon of salt. Spread out the potatoes and carrots in a single layer and roast for 15 minutes.

3. Meanwhile, rub the remaining 1 tablespoon of olive oil all over the cod. In a small bowl, combine the cumin, paprika, turmeric, and remaining ½ teaspoon of salt and sprinkle the mixture over the fish.

4. Remove the baking sheet from the oven and move the vegetables to clear four spots for the fish. Add the fish and red onion and roast for 15 to 20 minutes, until the fish is fully cooked and flakes easily with a fork. Garnish with parsley.

5. Refrigerate the leftovers in an airtight container for 3 to 4 days.

SUBSTITUTION TIP: Don't have russet potatoes? Use any kind of potato aside from sweet potatoes, which are a little too sweet. Replace 2 medium russet potatoes with 2 cups of chopped potato of a smaller variety such as red, yellow, or Yukon Gold.

Crab and Shrimp–Stuffed Avocados

Serves 4
Prep time: 20 minutes
5 or Fewer Ingredients

If you like to sleep in on the weekends and eat brunch instead of breakfast, this recipe is for you. You can whip up these absolutely scrumptious avocados the night before as long as you brush the cut edges with a little lemon juice and add a squeeze of citrus to the filling to prevent the avocados from oxidizing and turning brown. Cover them tightly in plastic wrap on a plate and store them in the refrigerator until you want to serve them.

4 avocados, pitted
½ pound crabmeat
½ pound cooked shrimp, peeled, deveined, and roughly chopped
1 red bell pepper, seeded and finely chopped
1 scallion, sliced on the bias
Salt
Freshly ground black pepper

Per serving: Calories: 462; Total Fat: 31g; Saturated Fat: 5g; Cholesterol: 163mg; Sodium: 806mg; Potassium: 1367mg; Magnesium: 116mg; Carbohydrates: 21g; Sugars: 3g; Fiber: 14g; Protein: 30g; Added Sugars: 0g; Vitamin K: 52mcg

1. Scoop out the center of the avocados, leaving a ½-inch layer of fruit in each half. Transfer the scooped-out portion to a large bowl and set the avocado halves aside.

2. Add the crabmeat, shrimp, bell pepper, and scallion to the bowl and mix well.

3. Season the filling with salt and pepper.

4. Spoon the seafood filling into the avocado halves and serve immediately.

5. Refrigerate the leftovers in an airtight container for 3 to 4 days.

PREP TIP: If you enjoy a creamier filling, add a couple tablespoons of mayonnaise or sour cream for a tangier flavor. Shredded carrot, minced red onion, and even chopped mango can take the filling to a sublime level. Experiment to find your favorite enhancements.

Fiery Salmon Skewers

Serves 4
Prep time: 10 minutes, plus 1 hour to marinate / Cook time: 15 minutes
Worth the Wait

Kebabs are fun to make and look so festive balanced on top of a colorful rice dish. Add a couple zucchini chunks, cherry tomatoes, mushrooms, or red onion pieces to the skewers to bulk up your meal. You can also create a couple veggie-only skewers to pair with your salmon ones.

¼ cup extra-virgin olive oil

Juice of 1 lime

2 teaspoons minced garlic

1 teaspoon ground cumin

½ teaspoon paprika

½ teaspoon of cayenne pepper

1 pound skinless salmon fillet, cut into 1-inch pieces

1 large red onion, cut into 1-inch chunks

8 wood skewers, soaked for 30 minutes

¼ cup roughly chopped fresh cilantro

1. In a medium bowl, stir together the olive oil, lime juice, garlic, cumin, paprika, and cayenne.

2. Add the salmon pieces and the red onion and toss to coat.

3. Place the bowl in the refrigerator for 1 hour to marinate.

4. Preheat the oven to 400°F.

5. Thread the salmon onto the skewers and place them on a baking sheet.

6. Roast the kebabs in the oven, turning once, until the fish flakes easily when pressed, 10 to 12 minutes total.

7. Garnish with chopped cilantro and serve.

8. Refrigerate the leftovers in an airtight container for 3 to 4 days.

Per serving: Calories: 242; Total Fat: 14g; Saturated Fat: 2g; Cholesterol: 62mg; Sodium: 53mg; Potassium: 653mg; Magnesium: 41mg; Carbohydrates: 5g; Sugars: 2g; Fiber: 1g; Protein: 23g; Added Sugars: 0g; Vitamin K: 8mcg

PREP TIP: If you own a barbecue grill and the weather is favorable, grill these kebabs for a lovely smoky flavor. Be sure to soak the wood skewers so they don't catch fire. Alternatively, you can use metal skewers. Baste the kebabs with the remaining marinade and grill them for about 8 minutes total, turning at least once.

Zucchini Linguine and White Clam Sauce

QUICK

Serves 4
Prep time: 10 minutes / Cook time: 15 minutes

Zucchini noodles keep this dish lower in carbs but still as satisfying as a pasta meal. The clams provide plenty of protein.

3 tablespoons extra-virgin olive oil, divided
3 garlic cloves, minced
1 shallot, sliced
Kosher salt
Freshly ground black pepper
24 littleneck clams, soaked in cold water for 10 minutes, drained, and scrubbed
½ cup dry white wine
3 zucchini, spiralized or cut into ribbons
1 teaspoon red pepper flakes
½ cup grated Parmesan cheese
½ cup chopped fresh parsley, lightly packed

Per serving: Calories: 274; Total Fat: 15g; Saturated Fat: 4g; Cholesterol: 37mg; Sodium: 805mg; Potassium: 526mg; Magnesium: 55mg; Carbohydrates: 12g; Sugars: 4g; Fiber: 2g; Protein: 19g; Added Sugars: 0g; Vitamin K: 135mcg

1. In a large, heavy pot, heat 2 tablespoons of olive oil over medium heat. Add the garlic and shallot. Season with salt and pepper and cook for 1 to 2 minutes, until fragrant.

2. Add the clams and wine. Cover and cook until the clams open, about 10 minutes. Remove the clams with all the liquid and set aside in a large bowl.

3. Wipe down the emptied pot and heat the remaining 1 tablespoon of oil over medium heat. Once the oil is warm, add the zucchini ribbons. Cook for about 3 minutes. Add the red pepper flakes and Parmesan cheese. Stir until the cheese is melted.

4. Turn off the heat and add the clams and liquid back to the pot. Toss to combine and transfer to a large serving bowl. Sprinkle with the fresh parsley and serve immediately.

5. Refrigerate the leftovers in an airtight container for up to 2 days.

SUBSTITUTION TIP: In place of fresh clams, you can use 1 (15-ounce) can of chopped clams. Skip step 2 and instead of adding the whole clams in step 4, add the canned clams with their juice.

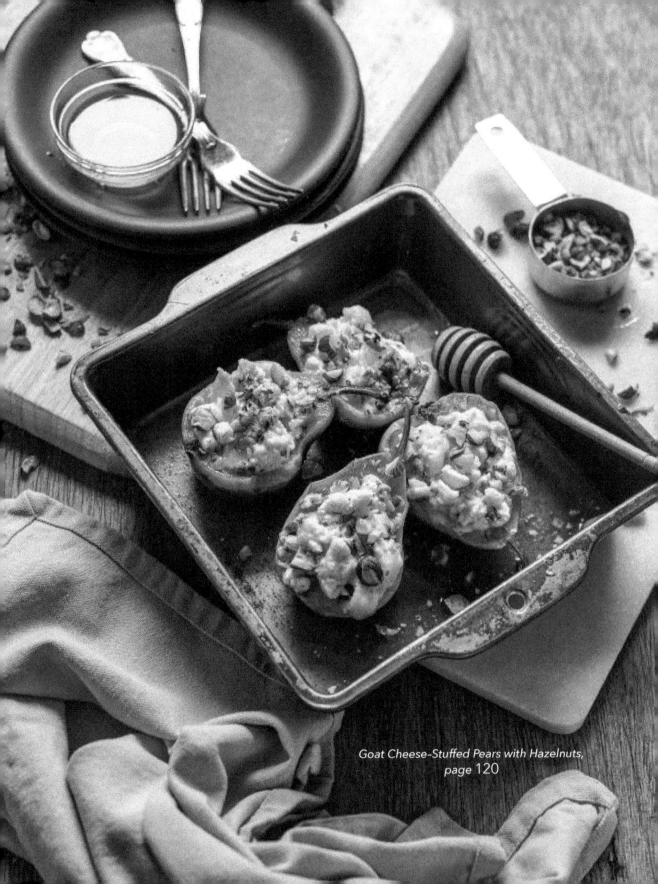

Goat Cheese-Stuffed Pears with Hazelnuts,
page 120

Chapter 7

Desserts

Goat Cheese–Stuffed Pears with Hazelnuts

Serves 4
Prep time: 5 minutes / Cook time: 20 minutes
5 or Fewer Ingredients

Some desserts seem to be better suited to certain seasons even if they can be eaten year-round. This recipe is a fall dessert: a dish for when the air is crisp and the trees are just starting to change color. The first creamy bite, tangy and rich with a hint of sweetness, will remind you of decadent cheesecake but it is actually quite healthy. Pears add dietary fiber, and the blend of goat cheese and tofu keeps this dessert lower in saturated fats.

1 tablespoon extra-virgin olive oil
2 ripe medium pears, halved lengthwise, cored and hollowed out with a spoon
½ cup water
4 tablespoons goat cheese
2 ounces firm tofu
2 tablespoons honey
¼ cup roughly chopped hazelnuts

1. Preheat the oven to 350°F.

2. In a medium skillet, heat the olive oil over medium heat.

3. Place the pears in the skillet, skin-side up, and lightly brown them, about 2 minutes.

4. Place the pears in an 8 x 8-inch square baking dish, hollow-side up, and pour the water into the baking dish, taking care not to get any in the hollow part of the pears.

5. Roast the pears until softened, about 10 minutes. Remove the pears from the oven.

6. Mash together the goat cheese and tofu until well combined. Then stir in the honey and hazelnuts.

7. Evenly divide the goat cheese mixture among the four pear halves and put them back in the oven for 5 minutes.

8. Serve warm. Refrigerate the leftovers in an airtight container for 3 to 4 days.

PREP TIP: Pears are one of those fruits that seem to bruise easily in the bag on the way home from the grocery store, so be gentle. Place your pears in a bowl at room temperature until the skin by the stem yields a little when pressed lightly. If you need them to ripen faster, place them in a paper bag.

Per serving: Calories: 197; Total Fat: 11g; Saturated Fat: 2g; Cholesterol: 3mg; Sodium: 36mg; Potassium: 193mg; Magnesium: 28mg; Carbohydrates: 24g; Sugars: 9g; Fiber: 4g; Protein: 5g; Added Sugars: 9g; Vitamin K: 7mcg

Spiced Oranges with Dates

Serves 4
Prep time: 15 minutes
5 or Fewer Ingredients

Desserts don't have to be elaborate creations full of sugar and saturated fats; the end of your meal can be light and simple. One orange contains the minimum recommended daily amount of vitamin C for an adult and is also a wonderful source of vitamin A, limonoid, iron, and calcium. Citrus can help boost your immune system, combat the common cold, and lower cholesterol.

4 large oranges
2 large blood oranges
  or cara cara oranges
¼ cup coarsely
  chopped
  Medjool dates
⅛ teaspoon ground
  cloves
2 tablespoons chopped
  hazelnuts

1. Use a sharp paring knife to cut the skin and pith off the oranges so you have just the flesh. Follow the membranes to cut out the sections of the oranges, and place them in a medium bowl. Squeeze any remaining juice from the membranes into the bowl with the fruit.

2. Add the dates, cloves, and hazelnuts to the bowl and toss to combine.

3. Serve spooned into individual bowls.

4. Prep in advance or store leftovers by refrigerating in an airtight container for 3 to 5 days.

PREP TIP: Blood oranges are usually in season from early winter to spring, so that is the time they will be most affordable. Look for oranges that feel firm and heavy for their size because that indicates that the fruit is juicy. Ripe blood oranges can have a little green tint to the rind, but this will not affect their taste.

Per serving: Calories: 178; Total Fat: 3g; Saturated Fat: 0g; Cholesterol: 0mg; Sodium: 0mg; Potassium: 584mg; Magnesium: 37mg; Carbohydrates: 40g; Sugars: 32g; Fiber: 8g; Protein: 3g; Added Sugars: 0g; Vitamin K: 1mcg

Protein-Packed Chocolate Mousse

VEGETARIAN

Serves 4
Prep time: 10 minutes, plus 30 minutes to chill

Tofu is an easy way to sneak in some protein when it comes to desserts. That's because tofu takes on the flavor of all the other ingredients. When you make this mousse, you just may feel like the ultimate sneaky chef.

¼ cup semisweet
  chocolate chips
⅔ cup unsweetened
  soy milk
½ (16-ounce) package
  silken tofu
½ cup cocoa powder
2 teaspoons honey
2 teaspoons vanilla
  extract
Berries of your choice,
  for garnish (optional)
Fresh mint, for garnish
  (optional)
Shaved chocolate, for
  garnish (optional)

1. Melt the chocolate chips on the stove using a double boiler or in the microwave in a microwave-safe bowl.

2. In a food processor or blender, combine the soy milk, tofu, cocoa powder, honey, and vanilla. Transfer the melted chocolate to the food processor and blend until smooth.

3. Scoop the mixture into four dishes. Refrigerate for 30 minutes. To serve, garnish with berries (if using), mint (if using), and shaved chocolate (if using).

4. Prep in advance or store leftovers by refrigerating them in an airtight container for up to 4 days.

PREP TIP: Using silken tofu will you give you more of a pudding consistency. If you want a thicker mousse, use firm or extra-firm tofu.

Per serving: Calories: 136; Total Fat: 7g; Saturated Fat: 3g; Cholesterol: 1mg; Sodium: 23mg; Potassium: 442mg; Magnesium: 86mg; Carbohydrates: 16g; Sugars: 5g; Fiber: 4g; Protein: 7g; Added Sugars: 3g; Vitamin K: 2mcg

Oatmeal Dark Chocolate Chip Peanut Butter Cookies

VEGETARIAN
QUICK

Makes 24
Prep time: 15 minutes / Cook time: 10 minutes

These chocolate chip cookies include wholesome ingredients like peanut butter, rolled oats, and dark chocolate chips. Bake them for 8 minutes for a chewy, soft cookie or for 10 minutes for a crispy cookie. The choice is yours. Either way, they make the perfect guilt-free dessert.

1½ cups natural creamy peanut butter
½ cup dark brown sugar
2 large eggs
1 cup old-fashioned rolled oats
1 teaspoon baking soda
½ teaspoon salt
½ cup dark chocolate chips

1. Preheat the oven to 350°F. Line a baking sheet with parchment paper.

2. In the bowl of a stand mixer fitted with the paddle attachment, whip the peanut butter until very smooth. Continue beating and add the brown sugar and then one egg at a time, until fluffy. Beat in the oats, baking soda, and salt until combined. Fold in the dark chocolate chips.

3. Use a small cookie scoop or teaspoon to place spoonfuls of the cookie dough on the baking sheet, about 2 inches apart. Bake for 8 to 10 minutes depending on your preferred level of doneness.

4. Store at room temperature in an airtight container for up to 7 days.

PREP TIP: For a fluffier cookie, refrigerate the dough for 30 minutes before baking.

SUBSTITUTION TIP: Try raisins instead of the chocolate chips.

Per serving (1 cookie): Calories: 156; Total Fat: 11g; Saturated Fat: 2g; Cholesterol: 16mg; Sodium: 110mg; Potassium: 171mg; Magnesium: 59mg; Carbohydrates: 12g; Sugars: 1g; Fiber: 2g; Protein: 5g; Added Sugars: 5g; Vitamin K: 0mcg

Melon-Lime Sorbet

Serves 8
Prep time: 15 minutes, plus 4 to 6 hours to freeze and 30 minutes to set
5 or Fewer Ingredients

You do not need an ice cream maker to create perfect sorbets and sherbets, just a bit of imagination and patience. Homemade sorbet contains very little added sugar and tons of fruit. You can certainly sweeten it up, but very ripe melons might allow you to skip the honey altogether. Serve your sorbet with a dollop of whipped coconut cream and a sprig of fresh spearmint.

1 small honeydew melon, peeled, seeded, and cut into 1-inch chunks
1 small cantaloupe, peeled, seeded, and cut into 1-inch chunks
2 tablespoons honey
2 tablespoons freshly squeezed lime juice
Pinch cinnamon
Water as needed

1. Spread the honeydew and cantaloupe out on a baking sheet lined with parchment paper. Place the baking sheet in the freezer for 4 to 6 hours until the fruit is frozen.

2. In a food processor, combine the frozen melon chunks, honey, lime juice, and cinnamon.

3. Pulse until smooth, adding water (a tablespoon at a time) if needed to puree the melon.

4. Transfer the mixture to a resealable container and place it in the freezer until set, about 30 minutes.

5. Freeze in an airtight "freezer" container for up to 1 month.

PREP TIP: Almost any fruit will work in this recipe. You can try watermelon, peaches, plums, mangos, or berries. Some fruits have more water in them than others, so if you're using produce that's less juicy, add extra water or apple juice to create a smooth puree.

Per serving: Calories: 81; Total Fat: 0g; Saturated Fat: 0g; Cholesterol: 0mg; Sodium: 32mg; Potassium: 439mg; Magnesium: 20mg; Carbohydrates: 21g; Sugars: 15g; Fiber: 2g; Protein: 1g; Added Sugars: 4g; Vitamin K: 5mcg

Coconut Date Energy Bites

Makes 15
Prep time: 10 minutes
5 or Fewer Ingredients

These coconut date morsels are called "energy bites" because of their powerhouse nutrition profile. They contain protein and heart-healthy fats for a satisfying on-the-go snack that is in line with the DASH diet.

12 pitted
  Medjool dates
½ cup unsweetened
  shredded coconut
½ cup chopped
  walnuts or almonds
1½ tablespoons melted
  coconut oil

Place the dates, coconut, walnuts, and coconut oil in a food processor and pulse until the mixture becomes a paste. Form 2-inch bites, place in an airtight container, and store in the refrigerator for up to 2 weeks.

PREP TIP: After processing the mixture and before forming it into bites, refrigerate it for 30 minutes to make the bites easier to roll.

SUBSTITUTION TIP: Add a scoop of protein powder to the mixture, if desired. Also, instead of using the walnuts or in addition to them, try a variety of mix-ins like oats, peanut butter, mini dark chocolate chips, or raisins to make these energy bites into more of a treat.

Per serving (1 ball): Total Calories: 110; Total Fat: 6g; Saturated Fat: 3g; Cholesterol: 0mg; Sodium: 1mg; Potassium: 151mg; Total Carbohydrate: 16g; Fiber: 2g; Sugars: 13g; Protein: 1g

Fruit-Topped Meringues

Makes 24 cookies
Prep time: 15 minutes, plus 1 hour cooling time / Cook time: 50 minutes
5 or Fewer Ingredients
Worth the Wait

Meringues' crunchy exterior and delicately sweet melt-in-the-mouth interior make a perfect base for raspberries, which are full of essential vitamins and a good source of beta-carotene. They can promote healthy skin and reduce the risk of heart disease.

4 large egg whites, at room temperature
¼ teaspoon cream of tartar
Pinch salt
½ cup honey
1 cup raspberries

1. Preheat the oven to 200°F. Line two baking sheets with parchment paper and set aside.

2. In a large stainless steel bowl, beat the egg whites until they are frothy.

3. Beat in the cream of tartar and salt until soft peaks form, 4 to 5 minutes.

4. Beat in the honey, 1 tablespoon at a time, until stiff glossy peaks form.

5. Spoon the meringue batter onto the baking sheets using a tablespoon and create a small well in the center of each with the back of a spoon.

6. Bake until firm, 45 to 50 minutes. Turn off the heat and prop the door open to cool the meringues in the oven for at least 1 hour.

7. Refrigerate in an airtight container for up to 1 week and serve with a raspberry in the center of each meringue.

Per serving (2 meringues): Calories: 54; Total Fat: 0g; Saturated Fat: 0g; Cholesterol: 0mg; Sodium: 32mg; Potassium: 52mg; Magnesium: 4mg; Carbohydrates: 13g; Sugars: 0g; Fiber: 1g; Protein: 1g; Added Sugars: 12g; Vitamin K: 1mcg

Individual Apple Pockets

VEGETARIAN

QUICK

Serves 6
Prep time: 5 minutes / Cook time: 15 minutes

This is a delicious dessert or snack you can enjoy when cutting down on sugar. Each serving contains no more than 2 teaspoons of added sugars, meeting the American Heart Association Guidelines for heart-healthy desserts. And it has a decadent appeal: You can see the melted brown sugar and cinnamon glistening on the apple slices in each pocket.

1 organic puff pastry, rolled out, at room temperature
1 Gala apple, peeled and sliced
¼ cup brown sugar
⅛ teaspoon ground cinnamon
⅛ teaspoon ground cardamom
Nonstick cooking spray
Honey, for topping

1. Preheat the oven to 350°F.

2. Cut the pastry dough into four even discs.

3. In a small bowl, toss the apple slices with the brown sugar, cinnamon, and cardamom.

4. Spray a muffin tin very well with cooking spray. Be sure to spray only the muffin holders you plan to use.

5. Once sprayed, line the bottom of the muffin tin with the dough and place 1 or 2 broken apple slices on top. Fold the remaining dough over the apple and drizzle with honey.

6. Bake for 15 minutes or until brown and bubbly.

7. Store at room temperature in an airtight container for up to 2 days.

SUBSTITUTION TIP: For a gluten-free version of this dessert, use gluten-free puff pastry, which can be found online or at some grocery stores.

Per serving: Calories: 276; Total Fat: 16g; Saturated Fat: 4g; Cholesterol: 0mg; Sodium: 105mg; Potassium: 70mg; Magnesium: 9mg; Carbohydrates: 32g; Sugars: 3g; Fiber: 1g; Protein: 3g; Added Sugars: 9g; Vitamin K: 7mcg

Key Lime Cherry "Nice" Cream

DAIRY-FREE
VEGETARIAN
QUICK

Serves 4
Prep time: 10 minutes
5 or Fewer Ingredients

"Nice" cream is a trendy version of ice cream that doesn't require cream, nor does it require churning or any special ice cream equipment. The basis of the recipe is frozen banana, and any fruit, citrus, spices, and extracts can be added to give the nice cream unique flavors. Simply blend the ingredients in a food processor and enjoy a frozen treat.

4 frozen bananas, peeled
1 cup frozen dark sweet cherries
Grated zest and juice of 1 lime, divided
½ teaspoon vanilla extract
¼ teaspoon salt

1. Place the bananas, cherries, lime juice, vanilla, and salt in a food processor and puree until smooth, scraping the sides as needed.

2. Transfer the nice cream to bowls and top with the lime zest.

3. For leftovers, place the nice cream in airtight containers and store in the freezer for up to 1 month. Let it thaw for 30 minutes, until it reaches a soft-serve ice cream texture, before serving.

PREP TIP: Peel and slice ripe bananas and place them in a sealed plastic bag before freezing them. It is very hard to peel frozen bananas.

SUBSTITUTION TIP: You can omit the salt from this recipe if you need to. Another variation is to try blueberries and lemon instead of the cherries and lime.

Per serving: Calories: 134; Total Fat: 0g; Saturated Fat: 0g; Cholesterol: 0mg; Sodium: 147mg; Potassium: 522mg; Magnesium: 37mg; Carbohydrates: 34g; Sugars: 20g; Fiber: 4g; Protein: 2g; Added Sugars: 0g; Vitamin K: 2mcg

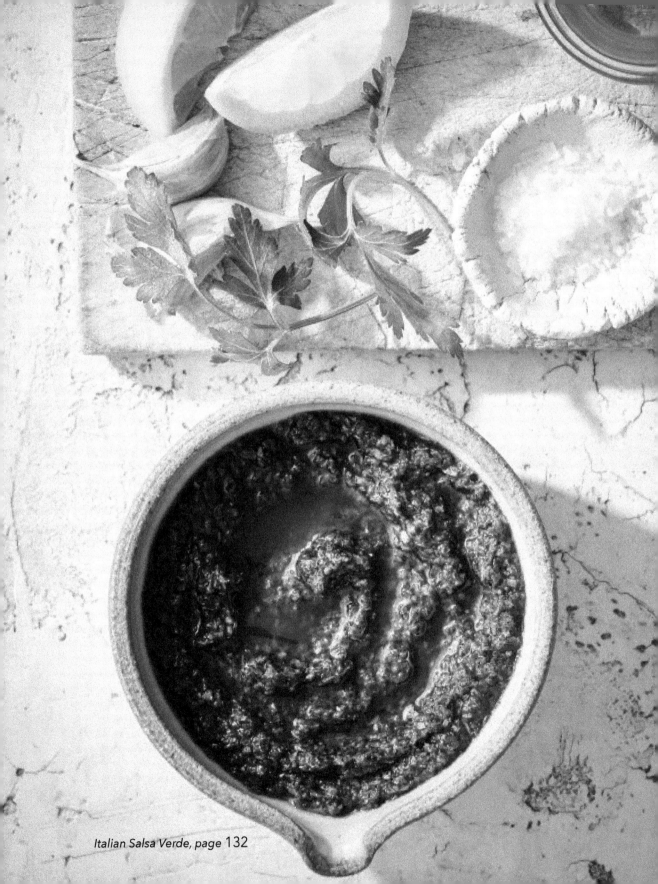

Italian Salsa Verde, page 132

Chapter 8

Staples

Italian Salsa Verde

Serves 6
Prep time: 10 minutes
5 or Fewer Ingredients

Italian salsa verde is a green sauce made with herbs, not to be confused with Mexican salsa verde, which is made with tomatillos. Traditionally, these ingredients would be hand-chopped, but you can use a food processor for convenience. This sauce is lovely on steak, fish, and egg dishes.

1 or 2 cups loosely packed fresh flat-leaf parsley
¼ cup extra-virgin olive oil
2 garlic cloves, peeled
½ teaspoon grated lemon zest plus 1 teaspoon freshly squeezed lemon juice
1 teaspoon white wine vinegar
1 teaspoon anchovy paste
½ teaspoon salt
¼ teaspoon freshly ground black pepper

1. In a food processor, combine the parsley, olive oil, garlic, lemon zest and juice, vinegar, anchovy paste, salt, and pepper and blend until smooth.

2. Refrigerate in an airtight container for up to 3 days.

SUBSTITUTION TIP: You can swap out the anchovy paste for 1 teaspoon of capers, which also add a bold and salty flavor. Capers are a more common kitchen staple and you may find you can use them more often than anchovies. Also, capers pair well with smoked salmon and are great for sprinkling onto your fish and into your salads.

Per serving: Calories: 86; Total Fat: 9g; Saturated Fat: 1g; Cholesterol: 1mg; Sodium: 224mg; Potassium: 65mg; Magnesium: 6mg; Carbohydrates: 1g; Sugars: 0g; Fiber: 0g; Protein: 1g; Added Sugars: 0g; Vitamin K: 169mcg

Roasted Red Pepper Dip

DAIRY-FREE
VEGETARIAN

Serves 6
Prep time: 10 minutes, plus 1 hour to chill / Cook time: 45 minutes
5 or Fewer Ingredients
Worth the Wait

Red bell peppers are packed with vitamin C and make a powerfully flavored dip. Many Mediterranean countries enjoy some type of red pepper dip as part of their cuisine. You can also use this recipe as a delectable sandwich spread.

**4 large red bell
peppers, seeded and
quartered**
1 large onion, chopped
**2 tablespoons
extra-virgin olive oil**
**1 teaspoon red wine
vinegar**
1½ teaspoons salt
**¼ teaspoon freshly
ground black pepper**
2 garlic cloves, peeled

Per serving: Calories: 85;
Total Fat: 5g; Saturated
Fat: 1g; Cholesterol: 0mg;
Sodium: 587mg; Potassium:
272mg; Magnesium: 16mg;
Carbohydrates: 9g; Sugars: 6g;
Fiber: 3g; Protein: 1g; Added
Sugars: 0g; Vitamin K: 8mcg

1. Preheat the oven to 425°F. Line a rimmed baking sheet with aluminum foil.

2. In a large bowl, toss the bell peppers and onion with the olive oil, vinegar, salt, and black pepper.

3. Spread out the peppers and onion in a single layer on the prepared baking sheet. Roast for 30 minutes; then add the garlic cloves and roast for 15 minutes more, until the peppers start to blacken on the edges. Remove from the oven and set aside to cool.

4. Transfer the contents of the baking sheet, including the oil, to a food processor or blender. Process until smooth.

5. Transfer to a bowl, cover, and refrigerate for 1 hour before serving.

6. Refrigerate the leftovers in an airtight container for up to 3 days.

PREP TIP: For your convenience, you can find frozen crushed garlic in the freezer section at major retail markets. 1 cube = 1 clove = 1 teaspoon. Just swap the 2 cloves of fresh garlic for 2 cubes of the frozen garlic.

Greek Cucumber-Yogurt Dip/Tzatziki

Serves 6
Prep time: 15 minutes

Tzatziki is a ubiquitous side, sauce, dip, and condiment in Greece—and for good reason. The refreshing flavor profile is the ideal companion to almost any hot meal. Garlic, a staple in nearly every cuisine in the world, adds a satisfying pungency. When purchasing garlic, choose heads that feel heavy for their size to ensure the cloves aren't dried out.

½ English cucumber, peeled and grated
2 cups low-fat plain Greek yogurt
3 tablespoons extra-virgin olive oil
Juice of 1 lemon
1 garlic clove, minced
2 tablespoons chopped fresh dill
1 or 2 teaspoons salt
1 teaspoon freshly ground black pepper
1 or 2 teaspoons red wine vinegar

1. Place the grated cucumber in a clean kitchen towel and twist the towel to squeeze out excess liquid; then place the cucumber in a large bowl.

2. Add the yogurt, olive oil, lemon juice, garlic, dill, salt, pepper, and vinegar and stir until well combined.

3. Taste and adjust the seasoning before serving. If desired, refrigerate the tzatziki for a bit before serving it to allow the flavors to mellow.

4. Refrigerate in an airtight container for up to 4 days.

PREP TIP: Be sure to squeeze out as much liquid from the grated cucumber as possible or your tzatziki may end up watery.

Per serving: Calories: 123; Total Fat: 8g; Saturated Fat: 2g; Cholesterol: 5mg; Sodium: 446mg; Potassium: 251mg; Magnesium: 22mg; Carbohydrates: 8g; Sugars: 6g; Fiber: 1g; Protein: 5g; Added Sugars: 0g; Vitamin K: 5mcg

Speedy Marinara Sauce

VEGETARIAN
QUICK

Makes 4 cups
Prep time: 5 minutes / Cook time: 25 minutes
5 or Fewer Ingredients

This marinara sauce is garlicky, rich, and packed with fresh herb flavor. Tomatoes owe their gorgeous red color to an antioxidant called lycopene, which can reduce the risk of several types of cancer, such as bladder, breast, lung, and prostate, as well as prevent heart disease. This antioxidant is hard for the body to digest when tomatoes are raw, so cooking the tomatoes in olive oil along with the other sauce ingredients can increase the absorption of the lycopene.

1 tablespoon extra-virgin olive oil
1 sweet onion, finely chopped
1 tablespoon minced garlic
2 (15-ounce) cans low-sodium crushed tomatoes
2 tablespoons chopped fresh basil
2 tablespoons chopped fresh oregano
Salt
Freshly ground black pepper

1. In a large saucepan, heat the olive oil over medium-high heat. Sauté the onion and garlic until softened and lightly caramelized, about 5 minutes.

2. Stir in the tomatoes and their juices and bring the mixture to a gentle boil. Reduce the heat to low and simmer, covered, for 15 to 20 minutes.

3. Remove the saucepan from the heat and stir in the basil and oregano. Season with salt and pepper. Serve immediately or refrigerate in an airtight container for up to 1 week.

STORAGE TIP: Basil often comes in large bunches, so you will probably have some left over. Wash and chop the basil and divide it among ice cube tray sections. Cover the herbs with water and freeze until firm. Pop the cubes out and transfer them to a freezer bag. When ready to use, add the entire ice cube to soups, sauces, and stews.

Per serving (½ cup): Calories: 36; Total Fat: 2g; Saturated Fat: 0g; Cholesterol: 0mg; Sodium: 31mg; Potassium: 229mg; Magnesium: 13mg; Carbohydrates: 5g; Sugars: 3g; Fiber: 2g; Protein: 1g; Added Sugars: 0g; Vitamin K: 7mcg

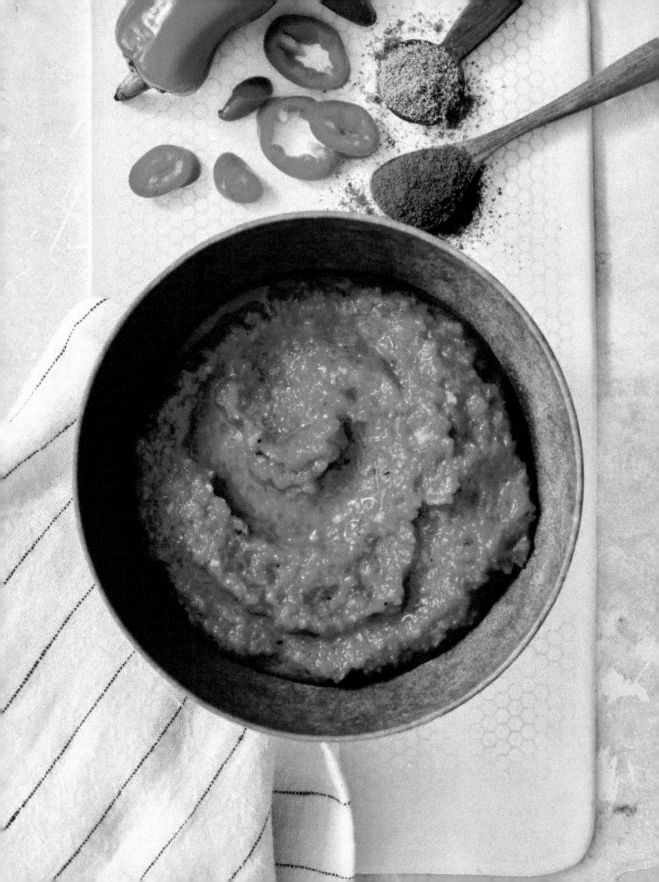

Harissa

DAIRY-FREE
VEGETARIAN
QUICK

Makes 1 cup
Prep time: 10 minutes / Cook time: 10 minutes

Harissa is a spicy North African paste made with roasted red bell peppers mixed with hot peppers and lots of spices. With vitamin C and various carotenoids, bell peppers benefit immunity, the skin, and eye health. Hot peppers contain capsaicin, an anti-inflammatory that may help relieve joint pain. Deliciously intense and rich in antioxidants, you may want to use harissa on everything.

2 tablespoons
extra-virgin olive oil

1 small red onion,
chopped

3 garlic cloves,
chopped

3 fresh red chiles,
seeded and chopped

1 (12-ounce) jar roasted
red peppers, drained

2 tablespoons freshly
squeezed lemon juice

1 tablespoon white
wine vinegar

½ teaspoon ground
coriander

½ teaspoon
ground cumin

½ teaspoon ground
caraway

½ teaspoon smoked
paprika

½ teaspoon salt

1 tablespoon
tomato paste

1. In a small skillet, heat the olive oil over medium heat. Add the onion, garlic, and chiles and cook for about 10 minutes, until caramelized.

2. Transfer the contents of the skillet to a food processor and add the roasted peppers, lemon juice, vinegar, coriander, cumin, caraway, paprika, salt, and tomato paste. Blend until smooth.

3. Refrigerate in an airtight container for up to 2 weeks.

Per serving (2 tablespoons): Calories: 57; Total Fat: 4g; Saturated Fat: 1g; Cholesterol: 0mg; Sodium: 250mg; Potassium: 175mg; Magnesium: 12mg; Carbohydrates: 6g; Sugars: 4g; Fiber: 1g; Protein: 1g; Added Sugars: 0g; Vitamin K: 7mcg

Simple Vinaigrette

Makes 1 cup
Prep time: 5 minutes
5 or Fewer Ingredients

A vinaigrette is really just a combination of an oil and an acid. This recipe uses extra-virgin olive oil and red wine vinegar, although you can use lemon juice for a bolder taste. Most store-bought dressings, even those that don't contain sugar, are made with a base of canola or soybean oil, which is pro-inflammatory and not nearly as tasty as olive oil. Stick with this healthier, money-saving option never buy bottled dressing again!

½ cup extra-virgin
   olive oil
¼ cup red wine vinegar
   or freshly squeezed
   lemon juice
1 tablespoon Dijon
   mustard
1 small garlic clove,
   finely minced
   (optional)
1 teaspoon dried herbs
   (oregano, rosemary,
   parsley, or thyme)
½ teaspoon salt
½ teaspoon freshly
   ground black pepper

In a glass mason jar with a lid, combine the olive oil, vinegar, mustard, garlic (if using), herbs, salt, and pepper and shake until well combined. Store in the refrigerator and bring to room temperature before serving. Be sure to shake the dressing well before using it as the oil and vinegar will naturally separate. Refrigerate in an airtight container for up to 2 weeks.

PREP TIP: If you prefer a creamy vinaigrette, add ½ cup of low-fat plain Greek yogurt to the mason jar and whisk until all the ingredients are well incorporated and develop a creamy texture.

Per serving (2 tablespoons): Calories: 122; Total Fat: 14g; Saturated Fat: 2g; Cholesterol: 0mg; Sodium: 168mg; Potassium: 8mg; Magnesium: 2mg; Carbohydrates: 0g; Sugars: 0g; Fiber: 0g; Protein: 0g; Added Sugars: 0g; Vitamin K: 9mcg

Seedy Crackers

Makes 24 crackers
Prep time: 25 minutes / Cook time: 15 minutes

These grain-free crackers satisfy a craving for something crunchy without compromising gut healing. Enjoy them topped with smoked salmon or a slice of avocado sprinkled with salt.

1 cup almond flour
1 tablespoon
  sesame seeds
1 tablespoon flaxseed
1 tablespoon
  chia seeds
¼ teaspoon
  baking soda
¼ teaspoon salt
Freshly ground black
  pepper
1 large egg, at room
  temperature

Per serving (6 crackers):
Calories: 199; Total
Fat: 16g; Saturated Fat: 2g;
Cholesterol: 47mg; Sodium:
248mg; Potassium: 234mg;
Magnesium: 95mg;
Carbohydrates: 8g; Sugars: 1g;
Fiber: 5g; Protein: 8g; Added
Sugars: 0g; Vitamin K: 0mcg

1. Preheat the oven to 350°F.

2. In a large bowl, combine the almond flour, sesame seeds, flaxseed, chia seeds, baking soda, salt, and pepper to taste and stir well.

3. In a small bowl, whisk the egg until well beaten. Add the beaten egg to the dry ingredients and stir well to combine and form the dough into a ball.

4. Place one layer of parchment paper on your countertop and place the dough on top. Cover with a second layer of parchment and, using a rolling pin, roll the dough to ⅛-inch thickness, aiming for a rectangular shape.

5. Cut the dough into 1- or 2-inch crackers and bake them on parchment until crispy and slightly golden, 10 to 15 minutes, depending on the thickness of the dough. Alternatively, you can bake the large rolled dough prior to cutting it and break it into free-form crackers once it is baked and crispy.

6. Refrigerate the crackers in an airtight container for up to 1 week.

SUBSTITUTION TIP: For variety, try this recipe using sunflower seeds instead of the flaxseed or chia. A budget-conscious swap, sunflower seeds are one of the least expensive options when it comes to buying nuts and seeds.

Tahini Sauce

Makes 2 cups
Prep time: 15 minutes
5 or Fewer Ingredients

Sesame seeds are a staple in Mediterranean cuisine and are used in all kinds of dishes, including tahini, which is used in hummus, savory dishes, and desserts such as halva. The pureed sesame seeds in tahini provide immunity-boosting minerals like copper and zinc.

3 garlic cloves, minced or mashed into a paste
½ cup tahini
½ cup freshly squeezed lemon juice
1 cup water
¼ teaspoon ground cumin
⅛ teaspoon salt

In a small bowl, whisk together the garlic, tahini, lemon juice, water, cumin, and salt until it develops into a smooth paste. Refrigerate in an airtight container for up to 1 month.

PREP TIP: Add parsley, cilantro, or Harissa (page 137) to add different flavors to this sauce. Tarator sauce is tahini sauce mixed with finely chopped fresh parsley. This sauce is popular drizzled over grilled fish or roasted vegetables.

Spiced Baked Pita Chips

Serves 6
Prep time: 10 minutes / Cook time: 10 minutes
5 or Fewer Ingredients

Pita bread is an essential part of daily life across most of the Mediterranean region. Pita makes a great vessel for eating plant-centric dips, such as basil pesto and Greek Cucumber-Yogurt Dip/Tzatziki (page 134).

2 tablespoons extra-virgin olive oil
1 teaspoon dried oregano
½ teaspoon paprika
½ teaspoon salt
¼ teaspoon freshly ground black pepper
¼ teaspoon cayenne pepper
3 pita breads, each cut into 8 triangles

1. Preheat the oven to 350°F. Line a rimmed baking sheet with parchment paper.

2. In a bowl, combine the olive oil, oregano, paprika, salt, black pepper, and cayenne. Mix well.

3. Spread out the pita triangles on the prepared baking sheet. Brush them with the oil mixture. Flip them over and brush the other sides.

4. Bake for 10 minutes, or until golden and crisp.

5. Store the pita chips at room temperature in an airtight container for up to 3 days.

SUBSTITUTION TIP: If you've got za'atar, it's a great choice for seasoning. Za'atar is a combination of oregano, thyme, sesame, and lemony sumac (and sometimes a bit of salt). It's perfect for flavoring pita. You can swap out the oregano and paprika in this recipe for 1½ teaspoons of this flavorful Middle Eastern spice blend.

Per serving: Calories: 124; Total Fat: 5g; Saturated Fat: 1g; Cholesterol: 0mg; Sodium: 355mg; Potassium: 44mg; Magnesium: 9mg; Carbohydrates: 17g; Sugars: 0g; Fiber: 1g; Protein: 3g; Added Sugars: 0g; Vitamin K: 4mcg

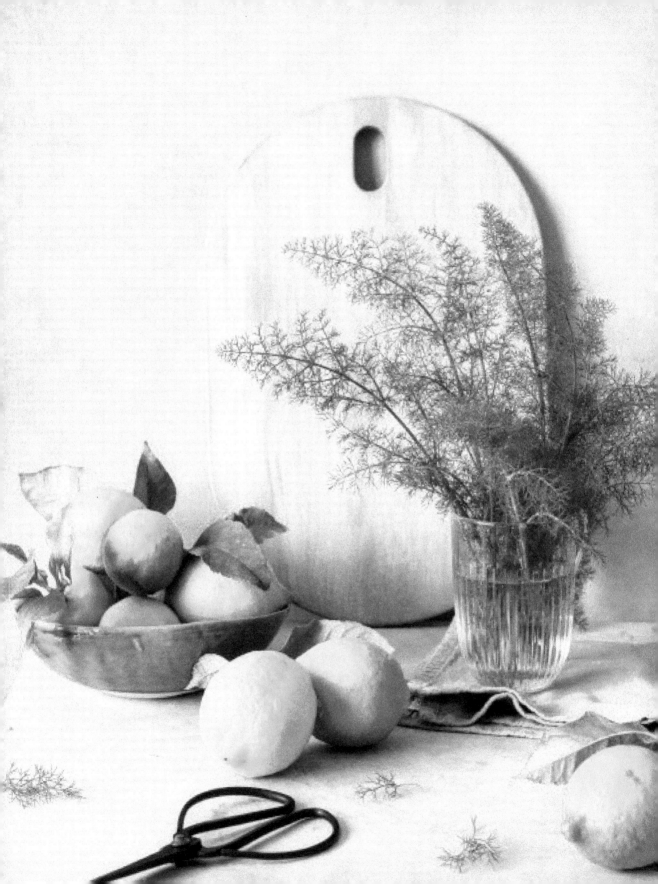

Measurement Conversions

Volume Equivalents (Liquid)

US STANDARD	US STANDARD (OUNCES)	METRIC (APPROX.)
2 tablespoons	1 fl. oz.	30 mL
¼ cup	2 fl. oz.	60 mL
½ cup	4 fl. oz.	120 mL
1 cup	8 fl. oz.	240 mL
1½ cups	12 fl. oz.	355 mL
2 cups or 1 pint	16 fl. oz.	475 mL
4 cups or 1 quart	32 fl. oz.	1 L
1 gallon	128 fl. oz.	4 L

Oven Temperatures

FAHRENHEIT (F)	CELSIUS (C) (APPROX.)
250°	120°
300°	150°
325°	165°
350°	180°
375°	190°
400°	200°
425°	220°
450°	230°

Volume Equivalents (Dry)

US STANDARD	METRIC (APPROX.)
⅛ teaspoon	0.5 mL
¼ teaspoon	1 mL
½ teaspoon	2 mL
¾ teaspoon	4 mL
1 teaspoon	5 mL
1 tablespoon	15 mL
¼ cup	59 mL
⅓ cup	79 mL
½ cup	118 mL
⅔ cup	156 mL
¾ cup	177 mL
1 cup	235 mL
2 cups or 1 pint	475 mL
3 cups	700 mL
4 cups or 1 quart	1 L

Weight Equivalents

US STANDARD	METRIC (APPROX.)
½ ounce	15 g
1 ounce	30 g
2 ounces	60 g
4 ounces	115 g
8 ounces	225 g
12 ounces	340 g
16 ounces or 1 pound	455 g

References

Alwarith, Jihad, Hana Kahleova, Lee Crosby, Alexa Brooks, Lizoralia Brandon, Susan M. Levin, and Neal D. Barnard. "The Role of Nutrition in Asthma Prevention and Treatment." *Nutrition Reviews* 78, no. 11 (2020): 928–38. doi.org/10.1093/nutrit/nuaa005.

Andreu-Reinón, María Encarnación, María Dolores Chirlaque, Diana Gavrila, Pilar Amiano, Javier Mar, Mikel Tainta, Eva Ardanaz, et al. "Mediterranean Diet and Risk of Dementia and Alzheimer's Disease in the EPIC-Spain Dementia Cohort Study." *Nutrients* 13, no. 2 (2021): 700. doi.org/10.3390/nu13020700.

Bailey, David G., George Dresser, and J. Malcolm O. Arnold. "Grapefruit–Medication Interactions: Forbidden Fruit or Avoidable Consequences?" *Canadian Medical Association Journal* 185, no. 4 (2012): 309–16. doi.org/10.1503/cmaj.120951.

Centers for Disease Control and Prevention. "Insulin Resistance and Diabetes." Centers for Disease Control and Prevention. August 10, 2021. cdc.gov/diabetes/basics/insulin-resistance.html.

de la Guía-Galipienso, Fernando, María Martínez-Ferran, Néstor Vallecillo, Carl J. Lavie, Fabian Sanchis-Gomar, and Helios Pareja-Galeano. "Vitamin D and Cardiovascular Health." *Clinical Nutrition* 40, no. 5 (2021): 2946–57. doi.org/10.1016/j.clnu.2020.12.025.

Esposito, Katherine, Maria Ida Maiorino, Giuseppe Bellastella, Paolo Chiodini, Demosthenes Panagiotakos, and Dario Giugliano. "A Journey into a Mediterranean Diet and Type 2 Diabetes: A Systematic Review with Meta-Analyses." *BMJ Open* 5, no. 8 (2015). doi.org/10.1136/bmjopen-2015-008222.

Hernáez, Álvaro, Albert Sanllorente, Olga Castañer, Miguel Á. Martínez-González, Emilio Ros, Xavier Pintó, Ramón Estruch, et al. "Increased Consumption of Virgin Olive Oil, Nuts, Legumes, Whole Grains, and Fish Promotes HDL Functions in Humans." *Molecular Nutrition & Food Research* 63, no. 6 (2019): 1800847. doi.org/10.1002/mnfr.201800847.

Kwok, T., P. Chook, M. Qiao, L. Tam, Y. K. Poon, A. T. Ahuja, J. Woo, D. S. Celermajer, and K. S. Woo. "Vitamin B-12 Supplementation Improves Arterial Function in Vegetarians with Subnormal Vitamin B-12 Status." *The Journal of*

Nutrition, Health & Aging 16, no. 6 (2012): 569–73. doi.org/10.1007/ s12603-012-0036-x.

Luo, Ming-Jie, Shan-Shan Rao, Yi-Juan Tan, Hao Yin, Xiong-Ke Hu, Yan Zhang, Yi-Wei Liu, et al. "Fasting before or after Wound Injury Accelerates Wound Healing through the Activation of Pro-Angiogenic SMOC1 and SCG2." *Theranostics* 10, no. 8 (2020): 3779–92. doi.org/10.7150/thno.44115.

Martín-Peláez, Sandra, Montse Fito, and Olga Castaner. "Mediterranean Diet Effects on Type 2 Diabetes Prevention, Disease Progression, and Related Mechanisms. A Review." *Nutrients* 12, no. 8 (2020): 2236. doi.org/10.3390/ nu12082236.

Mayo Clinic. "Dietary Fat: Know Which to Choose." Mayo Clinic. Healthy Lifestyle: Nutrition and Healthy Eating. April 8, 2021. mayoclinic.org/healthy-lifestyle/ nutrition-and-healthy-eating/in-depth/fat/art-20045550.

Mayo Clinic. "Red Wine and Resveratrol: Good for Your Heart?" Mayo Clinic. Mayo Foundation for Medical Education and Research. January 14, 2022. mayoclinic .org/diseases-conditions/heart-disease/in-depth/red-wine/art-20048281.

Mayo Clinic. "Water: How Much Should You Drink Every Day?" Mayo Clinic. Healthy Lifestyle: Nutrition and Healthy Eating. October 14, 2020. mayoclinic.org/ healthy-lifestyle/nutrition-and-healthy-eating/in-depth/water/art-20044256.

Mentella, Maria Chiara, Franco Scaldaferri, Caterina Ricci, Antonio Gasbarrini, and Giacinto Abele Donato Miggiano. "Cancer and Mediterranean Diet: A Review." *Nutrients* 11, no. 9 (2019): 2059. doi.org/10.3390/nu11092059.

Momoniat, Tasnim, Duha Ilyas, and Sunil Bhandari. "ACE Inhibitors and ARBs: Managing Potassium and Renal Function." *Cleveland Clinic Journal of Medicine* 86, no. 9 (2019): 601–7. doi.org/10.3949/ccjm.86a.18024.

O'Keefe, James H., Noel Torres-Acosta, Evan L. O'Keefe, Ibrahim M. Saeed, Carl J. Lavie, Sarah E. Smith, and Emilio Ros. "A Pesco-Mediterranean Diet with Intermittent Fasting: *JACC* Review Topic of the Week." *Journal of the American College of Cardiology* 76, no. 12 (2020): 1484–93. doi.org/ 10.1016/j.jacc.2020.07.049.

Palmer, Sharon. "Nutrients of Concern for Individuals Following a Plant-Based Diet." *Today's Dietitian*. June 2014. Accessed February 2, 2022. todaysdietitian .com/pdf/courses/PBDNutritentsofConcernPDF.pdf.

Pawlak, Roman. "Is Vitamin B$_{12}$ Deficiency a Risk Factor for Cardiovascular Disease in Vegetarians?" *American Journal of Preventive Medicine* 48, no. 6 (2015). doi.org/10.1016/j.amepre.2015.02.009.

Queiroz, Ana, Albertino Damasceno, Neusa Jessen, Célia Novela, Pedro Moreira, Nuno Lunet, and Patrícia Padrão. "Urinary Sodium and Potassium Excretion and Dietary Sources of Sodium in Maputo, Mozambique." *Nutrients* 9, no. 8 (2017). doi.org/10.3390/nu9080830.

Schwingshackl, Lukas, Jakub Morze, and Georg Hoffmann. "Mediterranean Diet and Health Status: Active Ingredients and Pharmacological Mechanisms." *British Journal of Pharmacology* 177, no. 6 (2019): 1241–57. doi.org/10.1111/bph.14778.

Sheps, Sheldon G. "Diuretics: A Cause of Low Potassium?" Mayo Clinic. Mayo Foundation for Medical Education and Research. April 21, 2020. mayoclinic.org/diseases-conditions/high-blood-pressure/expert-answers/blood-pressure/faq-20058432.

Sheps, Sheldon G. "Warfarin Diet: What Foods Should I Avoid?" Mayo Clinic. Mayo Foundation for Medical Education and Research. February 16, 2021. mayoclinic.org/diseases-conditions/thrombophlebitis/expert-answers/warfarin/faq-20058443.

Sizar, Omeed, Swapnil Khare, Radia T. Jamil, and Raja Talati. "Statin Medications." StatPearls [Internet]. U.S. National Library of Medicine. October 29, 2021. ncbi.nlm.nih.gov/books/NBK430940.

USDA. "Dietary Guidelines for Americans, 2020–2025." Accessed March 7, 2022. dietaryguidelines.gov/sites/default/files/2020-12/DGA_2020-2025_ExecutiveSummary_English.pdf.

U.S. News & World Report. "U.S. News Reveals Best Diet Rankings for 2022." Accessed February 2, 2022. usnews.com/info/blogs/press-room/articles/2022-01-04/u-s-news-reveals-best-diet-rankings-for-2022.

Index

Acknowledgments

I'd like to thank my dear friends Bridie Macdonald and Lisa Andrews for their continued support as my business has evolved. They have been there to cheer me on and support my accolades as a writer. I'd also like to thank my husband, JP, simply for being my rock. And props to my twins, Ailish and Julia, who have mirrored my joy of cooking and particularly excel in the art of pastries. It is my hope that they may someday open their "Duckling Café." And lastly, I'd like to thank my editor, Marjorie DeWitt, who has been such a joy to work with.

About the Author

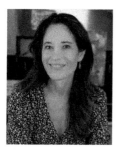

Lauren O'Connor, MS, RDN, is a registered dietitian, yoga instructor, and author of several books, including *Healthy Cooking for One* and *The Complete Healthy Eating Cookbook*. A member of the Academy of Nutrition and Dietetics (AND) and Food & Culinary Professionals (FCP), she received her master's degree in nutritional sciences from California State University, Los Angeles. She earned her culinary nutrition certification through Culinary Nutrition Studio, LLC. O'Connor has numerous mentions in major media outlets and has appeared on radio and TV. She writes for Livestrong and *Today's Dietitian* and contributes recipes and product reviews for *Food & Nutrition Magazine*.

O'Connor specializes in the dietary management of gastroesophageal reflux disease (GERD). She provides dietary and lifestyle practices to improve health outcomes for those with acid-reflux concerns. Learn more about her services at NutriSavvyHealth.com.

CPSIA information can be obtained
at www.ICGtesting.com
Printed in the USA
BVHW012357110423
662148BV00003B/14